Praise for the

The fight to maintain the NHS as a public service is one of the most fundamental battles we face today in our struggle for a British society that works for the many.

This wonderful, sobering book details how governments have teamed up with corporate and financial elites in an underhand effort to privatise and dismantle the NHS. Crucially, it also proposes solutions for how we can reclaim our NHS and the critical role of the grassroots groups leading this fight we can and must win.
Jeremy Corbyn, Leader of the Labour Party

Let's imagine something almost unimaginable. The leadership of a country with the world's finest health system, the pride of the nation, decides to dismantle it and replace it by the system that is by far the most costly, bureaucratic, and ineffective in the developed world, apparently under the influence of rigid doctrine (and perhaps greed). Unimaginable, but it appears to be happening, so Youssef El-Gingihy argues, all too persuasively, in his review of the steps being taken to convert the NHS to the failed US model.
Noam Chomsky

The Tories are remorseless in undermining the founding principles of the National Health Service. Youssef is a practising NHS doctor, who has seen the attacks at first hand. His book is an essential weapon in our fightback.
Ken Loach, Film director

The campaign to undermine the NHS is often concealed in Orwellian euphemisms. Dr Youssef El-Gingihy breaks through this web of deceit with this excellent primer of the who,what,

where and why your Health Service is being stolen from you.
John Pilger, investigative journalist and filmmaker

Like an increasing number of British doctors, El-Gingihy has gone through disbelief, anger and radicalisation at what he sees as the inexorable privatisation of our public health service..............
How to Dismantle the NHS in Ten Easy Steps (is) an attempt to translate the changes into plain English.......El-Gingihy's account is enlivened by his experience as a GP serving some of London's poorest patients
Richard Godwin, *Evening Standard*

How to Dismantle the NHS in 10 Easy Steps is a precise and devastating explanation of how a public health service - long the envy of the world - is furtively being dismembered for private, corporate gain by the likes of Virgin, Serco et al. The facts laid bare by El-Gingihy cry out for resistance. Arm yourself with this succinct book.
New Internationalist

Youssef El-Gingihy's accessible short book shows us why this attack on our most cherished public service is so important - a process that has been underway since the 1980s under Margaret Thatcher. Youssef provides a wealth of quite incredible information in 71 pages, so if you ever find yourself faced with a Tory offensive, you will be ready for the fight.And it's not just a Tory problem, El-Gingihy shows that every government over the past thirty years has contributed to the demise of the pride of the UK.

Nye Bevan, the creator of the service once said, 'The NHS will exist as long as there are folk left with the faith to fight for it.' El-Gingihy's book provides us with plenty of ammunition for that fight.
Cameron Panting, Counterfire

El-Gingihy is a GP in east London. His commitment to the NHS and the NHS ethos of compassion and caring shines through. Step by step, El-Gingihy takes us through the path to the destruction of the NHS, charted not just by the Tories but by New Labour as well. This book is an accessible account of the complexity of 25 years of attacks on the NHS, and tremendously valuable for that.
Gill George, *RS21 Magazine*

Packed with facts and figures, this shocking book reveals how the ruling class is dismantling our most precious institution, with impunity. At once infuriating and motivating, it is vital reading.
Feyzi Ismail

How to Dismantle the NHS in 10 Easy Steps

Second Edition

How to Dismantle the NHS in 10 Easy Steps

Second Edition

Youssef El-Gingihy

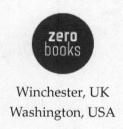

Winchester, UK
Washington, USA

JOHN HUNT PUBLISHING

First published by Zero Books, 2019
Zero Books is an imprint of John Hunt Publishing Ltd., No. 3 East St., Alresford,
Hampshire SO24 9EE, UK
office@jhpbooks.com
www.johnhuntpublishing.com
www.zero-books.net

For distributor details and how to order please visit the 'Ordering' section on our website.

ISBN: 978 1 78904 178 1
978 1 78904 179 8 (ebook)
Library of Congress Control Number: 2018949690

A CIP catalogue record for this book is available from the British Library.

Design: Stuart Davies

UK: Printed and bound by CPI Group (UK) Ltd, Croydon, CR0 4YY
US: Printed and bound by Thomson-Shore, 7300 West Joy Road, Dexter, MI 48130

We operate a distinctive and ethical publishing philosophy in
all areas of our business, from our global network of authors to
production and worldwide distribution.

Contents

Foreword to the Second Edition   1

Introduction   5

Step One: Create an Internal Market   9

Step Two: Introduce Public-Private Partnerships   11

Step Three: Facilitate the Corporate Takeover AKA
    Organise a Great Big Sell Off   20

Step Four: Install a Revolving Door   30

Step Five: Run A PR Smear Campaign   37

Step Six: Legislate for the Dismantling of the NHS   49

Step Seven: Plot against the NHS   64

Step Eight: Brew the Perfect Storm   70

Step Nine: Redesign the Workforce   78

Step Ten: Restructure the NHS into a US-style Insurance
    System   91

Afterword: How to Save the NHS in 5 Easy Steps   107

Reading List   115

References   116

DEDICATED TO ALL THOSE WHO HAVE FOUGHT FOR THE
NHS AND TO A FUTURE NHS FOR ALL TIME
I would like to thank those who showed the way and
illuminated my understanding of what has been happening to
our NHS. It is only through their contribution that I have been
able to write this book. All those years ago, they were lone
voices. More people are becoming aware of the marketisation
and privatisation of the NHS and are determined to fight
against vested interests to preserve it.

FOR ALI, AZZA AND JANA

Foreword to the Second Edition

'Events, dear boy, events,' as Prime Minister Harold Macmillan reportedly once said. Events have indeed overtaken the first edition of this book. The junior doctors' strike, the Conservative victory in the 2015 general election, the Corbyn phenomenon, the unexpected Brexit vote and the arguably even more unexpected loss of the Conservative majority in 2017.

As a medical student and junior doctor, I was largely unaware of what was happening to the NHS. The NHS is no longer a publicly provided and owned health system but instead has become a market system. It is in the process of becoming a two-tier system with the expansion of private healthcare insurance for those who can afford it and a third class US Medicaid style threadbare safety net for those who cannot.

My awakening came with the Health and Social Care Act 2012 under the Conservative led coalition government. I realised that the government and the mainstream media were not informing the public of the implications of these reforms. I decided to write this book in order to communicate to the public in concise, accessible terms what is really happening.

In the months that followed the publication of my book in 2015, I found myself embarking on a journey that I had scarcely even contemplated when I set out to write·it. Only weeks after publication, I was given a life-threatening diagnosis at the age of 34 and underwent several months of intensive treatment. Fortunately I went on to make a good recovery all thanks to the NHS. From fighting to save the NHS, the NHS saved my life. One dreads to think of the financial costs of such treatment in a private insurance system. A 2009 Harvard University study found that the majority of personal bankruptcies in the US - over a whopping 60 per cent - were due to healthcare costs.

At the outset of my illness, 50,000 junior doctors initiated strike action in protest at the government imposition of a new contract. It would turn out to be the largest industrial action of the twenty-first century in the UK. I even found myself thrust on to centre-stage in Parliament Square when I had the privilege of being invited to address the large crowds. Astonishingly I had received the first dose of my treatment the day before. I had expected to be laid up in bed that weekend; perhaps the mobilisation of my colleagues had served to invigorate me (I may have overdone it because things went downhill for the rest of that week!).

The junior doctor struggle was nothing less than living, breathing history being made even if it ended with a whimper rather than a bang. Of course, the lessons of this failure - some of them difficult to confront - must be evaluated if we are to rescue a publicly funded, provided, owned and accountable NHS. There have certainly been times when I have doubted my own analysis. One occasionally pauses to think that surely the government cannot be dismantling our precious, cherished NHS. Yet nostalgia will not be sufficient to salvage the NHS from the encroachment of market forces and the logic of capitalism. (Incidentally, the phrase - dismantling the NHS - appears to have entered the lexicon.)

One by one, I was saddened yet unsurprised to find my predictions coming true - the redesign of the workforce through the new junior doctor contract offering worse pay and conditions and the withdrawal of the student nursing bursary, the creation of economies of scale through chains of super hospitals and networks of GP surgeries ready for corporate takeover and the restructuring of the NHS into US-style accountable/integrated care organisations.

My journey has taken me from street demonstrations to the corridors of power in Westminster. I have met patients, campaigners, MPs, health correspondents, current as well as former civil servants, health ministers, shadow health teams and party leaders. What has perhaps impressed itself upon me most is how few have really grasped the direction of travel. I recall sitting in on a parliamentary Health Select Committee dismayed that nobody in the room appeared to fundamentally understand health economics or public health policy.

Policy has been concentrated in the upper echelons of the political, corporate and financial elite. This is a fundamental inheritance of the New Labour and Cameron eras. The culling of the civil service as a body of expertise has nullified institutional resistance. Instead, novice special advisers, often recruited from a tender age and seconded from corporate backgrounds, make up the backbone of the political party machines. The outsourcing of policy to think-tanks, the encirclement of Westminster by lobbyists, the revolving door and funding of the main parties all represent corporate capture of democracy and the privatisation of the state.

I met one former civil servant at the Department of Health, who resigned in disgust after seniors ignored her meticulously researched assessments because the minister would not want to see them. She confided to me that the term 'policy-based evidence making' was openly used inside the Department. In other words, evidence is tailored according to ideological policy rather than the use of evidence-based policy making.

The hollowing out of political parties, the mainstream media, the civil service and academia is one of the ghastly legacies of neoliberalism. It is necessary to rebuild the structures of civil society from the grassroots up. If history teaches us one thing, it is that only a broad-based mass movement can propel progress and save the NHS.

Yet the NHS cannot be preserved whilst the toxic effects of deregulated free market neoliberalism continue to be unleashed. Far reaching, progressive change of society - including public services run by staff, users and communities, a green

3

economy, the reversal of the death grip of financialisation, the democratisation of the economy, the dismantling of the offshore system as well as public investment and spending - will all be needed if we are to continue to have access to equitable, public healthcare.

When I wrote my book, I did so as a concerned doctor disturbed by a government ideologically fixated on privatisation against the wishes of the British people overwhelmingly in favour of the NHS. Since then, my unexpected illness has only reaffirmed my resolve to fight, alongside many others, to guarantee the provision of universal, comprehensive healthcare free at the point of need.

Introduction

I am a doctor. I work as a GP in London. Like most of you, I was born in a National Health Service hospital. I studied medicine and worked as a junior doctor in the NHS. I wrote this book because I fear that there will not be an NHS as our generation grows old and certainly not for our children. Yet the British public remains largely unaware of this and the media, with few exceptions, have failed in their duty to inform them. The remit of my book is charting how the NHS has been insidiously converted into a market-based healthcare system over the past 25 years. This process is accelerating under the Conservative government and the very existence of a National Health Service is in danger. This matters to all who use the NHS or are concerned by the privatisation of public services and the dismantling of equitable healthcare and welfare. The NHS - long the envy of the world - is being broken up into an insurance system based on the US model. Multinationals are opening the NHS oyster following on from the Health & Social Care Act (HSCA) 2012 and in preparation for the American model of accountable care. This is about much more than the NHS; it is about turbo-charged neoliberalism - the ideological doctrine that encompasses privatisation, financialisation, deregulation and shrinking the public sector.

Put simply, the next few years are likely to define whether the NHS continues to exist as a cherished institution or whether it is gradually dismantled into a privatised, insurance-based system. The issues at stake extend to the current neoliberal political and economic model and the kind of society we want to live in. It is likely to have huge ramifications for the direction Britain is heading in, at a time of great change, turmoil and chaos across the world.

NHS politics is an area that can be dry and foreboding to the public. The concept of this book is to make it accessible and to communicate clearly what is happening to our NHS. I want to shine a light on the deliberate destruction of the nation's most sacred institution whilst the majority of the British public have been kept in the dark by a neoliberal agenda pursued by the main political parties and the media. I only became aware of what was happening in 2011 at the time that the Health & Social Care Bill was making its way through Parliament. Incredibly, they don't really teach you much at medical school or as a junior doctor about how the NHS works and the history of its evolution. Maybe they should - there's certainly enough time in 5 years of studying.

Healthcare affects us and our loved ones arguably more than anything else in our lives. It would be a tragedy if the NHS were to be dismantled by vested interests - to great detriment to all of us - without the British public even having a say in the matter. People often feel impotent in the face of powerful interests. Yet the NHS belongs to us and we are the only ones who can fight for and save it.

Lots of questions are being asked of the NHS by politicians, the media and the public, such as:

- Can the NHS survive the current crisis?
- Is the NHS affordable?
- Where will the money come from?
- Would we be better off with universal private insurance?

I will try to answer them in this book. But what if these are the wrong questions diverting us from the real issues?

The National Health Service was created in 1948. It is one of the pillars of the welfare state. It was created as part of a planned economy to rebuild Britain after World War II. It is based on the principles of **universal, comprehensive, free healthcare** from cradle to grave with equity of care. It is part of our social fabric - 'a fundamental component of solidarity and equal citizenship'.[1]

The founder of the NHS, Aneurin Bevan, officially opened the first NHS hospital - Park Hospital in Manchester - on 5 July 1948. He met a 13-year-old girl with a liver condition by the name of Sylvia Diggory (née Beckingham), who became the first patient to be treated under the NHS. Ironically, the birthplace of the NHS, now renamed Trafford General, is one of many hospitals facing cuts and closures.[2]

Aneurin Bevan - a coal miner's son who fought hard against bitter opposition to establish the NHS - told her that it was a **'milestone in history - the most civilised step any country has ever taken'**. So, one day there was no such thing as the NHS and the next day it had come into existence. 1 April 2013 - the day the HSCA came into effect - represents the reversal of that process.

The HSCA is virtually impenetrable, but the main thrust of it is: Primary Care Trusts and Strategic Health Authorities have been disbanded. In their place, Clinical Commissioning Groups (CCGs) control about £60-80 billion of the NHS budget and commission local services. Commissioning often takes place through competitive tendering of NHS contracts open to the voluntary and private sectors. **But these recent events are the final stages in a journey that started over 30 years ago.**

Although nobody has told you this, the NHS has been effectively abolished. The national in National Health Service has been removed. It is fast becoming more of a notional health service subject to the whims of commissioners, cuts and rationing.

Now that may seem like a strange thing to say, seeing as you can still go to your local GP or hospital and receive free healthcare. On the surface, nothing seems to have changed. But, as you read on, you will discover that everything has. It will take many years for this to become apparent. The NHS lives on as a logo, which has helped to keep the public in the dark.

Our story really starts in the 1980s with Margaret Thatcher. Speaking at the sixtieth anniversary of the NHS in 2008, Kenneth

Clarke remarked that: 'In the late 1980s I would have said it is politically impossible to do what we are now doing.'[3]

Ken Clarke was talking about how the NHS has been gradually converted into a market-based healthcare system. After 30 years of neoliberalism, what was once impossible has become possible. Ken Clarke, of course, was there at the beginning. As health secretary under Thatcher, he got the ball rolling by introducing the internal market into the NHS in 1990.

Step One: Create an Internal Market

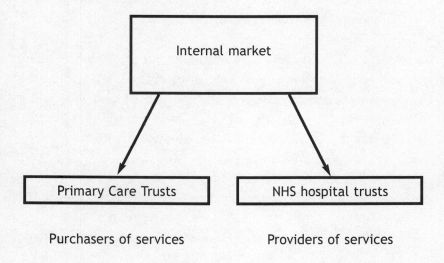

The 1980s saw the outsourcing of non-clinical hospital services such as catering, cleaning and laundry. Under John Major, most NHS bodies were made into trusts. NHS hospital trusts - or providers - run by boards of governors and chief executives 'sold' their services to purchasers, i.e. Primary Care Trusts. This became known as the purchaser-provider split. This means that hospitals have to compete against each other to get business. Except the NHS is not the City of London; what you really need in healthcare is collaboration rather than competition.

The internal market was introduced on the premise that the NHS is a monolithic bureaucracy, encased in red tape and stifled by centralisation. In other words, the public sector is inefficient and the private sector brings innovation. In fact, as a direct result of these reforms, NHS costs rose substantially. This is largely due to increased numbers of administrative and managerial staff.

A 2005 study by a team at York University demonstrated this.[1] Administrative costs rose from 5 per cent in the mid-1970s to 14 per cent in 2003 mainly due to internal market operations.

In fact, this study was commissioned by the Department of Health but hushed up, leading Parliament's Health Select Committee to state that they were 'dismayed' and 'appalled':

'The suspicion must remain that the DoH [Department of Health] does not want the full story to be revealed.'

The cost of running an internal NHS market has been estimated at between £4.5 to £10 billion a year.

Recent reforms have added to these costs. The HSCA could push these **administrative costs to 30 per cent. This would be similar to the US, where approximately 1 in 3 healthcare dollars are spent on administrative costs.**

This experience of market-based reforms has been borne out in other countries. A minority report from an NHS working group highlighted evidence from international experts of soaring administrative costs in New Zealand, Canada, Australia and Germany. In the case of Germany, these costs have soared by 63 per cent from 1992 to 2003 now accounting for 20 per cent of the health budget.[2]

Step Two: Introduce Public-Private Partnerships

The Private Finance Initiative (PFI) has been a fraud on the people.
Sir Howard Davies, chairman of RBS Bank

When Thatcher was asked what her greatest achievement had been, what was her answer?

a) Falklands War
b) Smashing the miners' strike and deunionisation
c) Privatisation of public utilities
d) The big bang deregulation of the City of London

None of these. It was... NEW LABOUR!

Ken Clarke, ever the good sport, was gracious enough to acknowledge the debt owed to New Labour for perpetuating the marketisation doctrines of Thatcherism. In fact, New Labour had pledged to abolish the internal market but then went full throttle in the opposite direction. New Labour's NHS Plan (2000) and NHS Improvement Plan (2004) resulted in the internal market expanding into an extensive market. This was again based on the premise that the private sector would introduce choice and competition as well as cutting costs.

In 2000, a 'concordat' between the NHS and private health firms paved the way for the provision of elective care and diagnostic tests, paid for by the NHS. This concordat facilitated private companies becoming permanent providers of treatment to NHS patients.

For example, when your GP requests an ultrasound or MRI scan, there is a good chance that a private company is being paid by the NHS to carry this out. Again, when your GP refers you to an outpatient clinic to see a specialist, this may be run by a private company. In theory, this sounds like a good idea.

Tim Evans, who negotiated the concordat on behalf of the private sector, looked forward **'to a time when the NHS would simply be a kitemark attached to the institutions and activities of a system of purely private providers'.**[1]

These public-private partnerships would take many shapes, the first of which were Independent Sector Treatment Centres (ISTCs). ISTCs served as the entry point for the private sector and were intended to 'unbundle' the high-volume, low-risk, lucrative NHS work, such as cataracts and knee and hip replacements. In so doing, they would reduce waiting times. The concept may have been simple enough but the reality was messy.[2]

As the British Medical Association (BMA) has shown, ISTC contracts were paid an average of 12 per cent more for each patient than the NHS tariff cost.[3] These sweeteners are often used in the outsourcing of public services to attract the private sector. They were also paid for a pre-determined number of cases - in bulk - regardless of whether procedures were carried out or not. To take one example, **'Netcare did not perform nearly 40% of the work it had been contracted to do,' receiving £35 million for patients it never treated.**[4]

As of 2010, an overall average of just 85 per cent of contracted activity was delivered. This ended up costing £5.6 billion over 5 years yet by 2008 barely exceeded 2 per cent of 8.6 million elective procedures.

Bringing in the private sector did not cut costs. It increased costs to the detriment of the NHS and patients, with only the private sector benefiting.

On top of this, clinical complications and legal costs were covered by the NHS. Yet more sugar-coating. There have also been repeated concerns about quality of care. Nevertheless, ISTCs were widened into the Extended Choice Network, which comprised 149 privately-run facilities by 2009.

Outsourced services are allowed to use the NHS logo meaning

that patients are in the dark about who exactly provides their care. It was win-win for ISTC contractors and lose-lose for the NHS and patients. So if you are having an elective procedure or operation in the future, find out if it is being performed by a private company.

ISTCs were small fry compared to Private Finance Initiatives (PFIs). New Labour expanded PFIs, originally dreamt up under John Major, to build *and run* infrastructure projects. PFI schemes were used to build roads, schools, prisons and hospitals. PFI hospitals made up the biggest chunk. These projects were put out to tender to PFI consortia of bankers, construction firms and facilities management companies. The argument went that Labour had inherited public services in a diabolical state of neglect. The mantra from on high was that there was no alternative to the private financing of whole swathes of infrastructure. This kept the money off the Treasury's books and was supposed to reduce the costs of government borrowing. As Alan Milburn - a former Labour health secretary described by *Private Eye* as an 'almost maniacal convert to PFI' - put it, 'It's PFI or bust.'

It was a persuasive argument and there were many seduced and dazzled by its lustre. The Blairite Third Way would somehow square the circle by delivering new schools, hospitals, roads, railways and prisons without the debt or inefficiency of the public sector. It seemed too good to be true. Yet at the time, very few seriously interrogated the small print of the contracts. Those who dared to question the orthodoxy *du jour* were conveniently swatted away.

As early as 1999, Richard Smith, then editor of the *British Medical Journal (BMJ)*, denounced it as *PFI: Perfidious Financial Idiocy* in an editorial revealing that the repayments would be exorbitant. In the same year, Professor Allyson Pollock and colleagues had published a paper sounding the alarm over the potential disastrous consequences of PFI debt and financialisation of public services. In a classic 2004 long read for *Private Eye* titled

P.F.Eye - An Idiot's guide to the Private Finance Initiative - the late Paul Foot exposed the seedy underbelly of its history.

It later transpired that the process of bringing in PFI had not exactly been transparent. As researcher and campaigner Joel Benjamin of *The People versus PFI* (full declaration I have made Joel's acquaintance in recent years) has written: 'Politicians did not simply wake up one morning and declare that banks should finance and own schools and hospitals, off-balance-sheet, via offshore tax havens, they were lobbied by City interests, prior to the implementation of PFI.'

A PFI panel was set up by Chancellor Ken Clarke in 1993. It mutated into a taskforce inside HM Treasury and was eventually rebranded as Partnerships UK. Partnerships UK employed a revolving door with secondments of various executives from big banks parachuted in. It was later privatised with the shares sold off to financial institutions including Barclays, HSBC and RBS. Public-private partnerships were also exported as a global model.

Now the unheeded prophesies of the Cassandras have come true. The completed PFI projects have been leased back to the government (or in the case of PFI hospitals, to NHS trusts) with repayments, usually over 25 to 30 years, at high interest rates (as high as 14 per cent). Repayments are indexed so that they increase every year, even when the income of NHS trusts is falling. The Conservatives are fond of drawing analogies between the economy and a household budget; so think of PFI as a mortgage...a hideously expensive mortgage, which ends up bankrupting the family!

The bill for hospitals alone is projected to rise above £79 billion. This exceeds the original capital cost (i.e. actual value) of £11.4 billion seven-fold.[5]

PFIs came with strings attached in which 'facilities maintenance' was also subcontracted out. For example, if you need to change a plug socket or a light bulb, only a specific contractor is allowed to do this.[6] A *Daily Telegraph* investigation flagged up several examples for the edification of the general public but this one really stands out:

One hospital was charged £52,000 for a job which should have cost £750.[7]

If you wanted to think up a way to bleed the NHS dry then you would struggle to do better than PFI. Is it any wonder then that **more than half of NHS hospitals are now in deficit and potentially in danger of going bust?[8]**

One of the main factors behind this is PFI, although this is not usually mentioned.

The total PFI tab for the taxpayer stands at over £300 billion for infrastructure projects with a capital worth of £54.7 billion.

That's a difference of approaching £250 billion.

Just think what you could do with this money?

Well it would pay for all the nurses (there are just under 350,000) in the NHS for 10 years.

Plus all 40,000 consultants for 10 years.

Plus all 40,000 GPs for 10 years.[9]

Still tens of billions to burn.

Well there are 18,000 surgeons in England. It costs around £400,000 to train a surgeon (surgeons and fighter pilots are the two most expensive professions to train so I'm told). So the next generation or two of surgeons, i.e. another 18,000, would cost around £7 billion.[10]

Plus 80 state of the art hospitals (based on the estimated cost of the new Papworth hospital - the national heart and lung transplant centre - at £165 million).[11]

And pay for chemotherapy and radiotherapy for a million cancer patients (at £35,000 each).[12]

If you wanted to keep it simple then the PFI drain would cover the entire NHS budget for over 2 years.

And with the leftover change, you could cover Alexis Sanchez's £600,000 a week salary should Manchester United ever require a government bail-out!

PFIs and ISTCs are just two examples of how the private sector and really a few high-net-worth individuals have siphoned off public money.

I was born at the Queen Elizabeth Hospital in Birmingham. My father has been under their excellent care for many years. It has been rebuilt as a PFI hospital with the original cost at £627 million but repayments will reach £2.58 billion.[13] This begs the question: how many other patients could receive fantastic NHS care for this money?

I did my GP training at the Royal London Hospital, which is part of Barts Health Trust. This is the largest trust in the country and accordingly has the most expensive PFI scheme, which is one of Innisfree's flagship projects. Innisfree - a fund management company in the City of London - is one of the biggest players in the PFI market.

As one comes out of Whitechapel tube station, the new Royal London Hospital certainly looks impressive. Its glistening blue tower is emblematic of an ultra-modern twenty-first century NHS. It looms over the ruins of the crumbling Victorian hospital made famous in David Lynch's film *The Elephant Man*. Up and down the country, this is the slick, corporate sheen of PFI hospitals. Inside, the first impression is that it is state of the art. Yet there is also an aesthetic and functional brutalism with labyrinthine corridors and sunless, windowless rooms. There are fewer junior doctor offices and overnight rooms. Intriguingly, PFI hospitals have been designed with significant numbers of individual rooms as opposed to conventional wards. This is clearly beneficial for patients and reduces the risk of transmission of infections. However, it suggests that privately financed hospitals are potentially anticipating something else - the expansion of private healthcare.

The original capital cost (i.e. actual value) of the Barts Health PFI was £1.1 billion (around £1 million per bed) but will end up costing £7.1 billion by 2049.[14] A total of **£6 billion will go to the PFI consortium Skanska Innisfree and partners.** Chairman of Imperial College Healthcare Sir Richard Sykes has previously pointed out that **Barts Health are paying £100 million a year in interest before they even see a patient.**[15] **That's £3 billion, just in interest, over 30 years. Imagine what you could do for healthcare in East London with this money.**

So it's not exactly surprising that Barts Health has declared that it is in dire financial straits. It was put into special measures by the Care Quality Commission in 2015. Its restructuring entailed redundancies for hundreds of staff and down-banding of others. Since I completed my GP training in Tower Hamlets, services have disappeared at an alarming rate. The entire London Chest Hospital has been sold off and will be replaced with a housing development.

The view from the Royal London cafeteria is direct on to the City of London. The irony of this vista is not lost on me. You could say it's a somewhat dyspeptic perspective for diners. At night, if you stand outside the hospital and crane your neck to the top floors, you will notice that they are permanently dark. These wards have been mothballed because the funding ran out.

The majority shareholder in Innisfree is Jersey-based Coutts & Co, which in turn is part of the RBS group. RBS was the biggest bank in the world by assets when it failed in 2008. The combined cost of the government bail-out and losses incurred since is over £100 billion or close to the NHS budget for one year. As campaigners see it, banks and other financial companies have used extortionate interest rates to boost their revenue from captive public services.

Banking leviathan HSBC also has a stake in PFI hospitals. It has even been described as owning outright three NHS hospitals. A provocative documentary titled *HSBC: Gangsters of Finance* pointed out that the bank has been caught red-handed laundering money for Mexican and Colombian drug cartels,

Russian gangsters and organisations linked to Al Qaeda. Campaigners argue that, with this unedifying track record, such corporate and financial interests should not be entrusted with hospitals and schools.

The Princess Royal Hospital in Bromley was another Innisfree gift to the taxpayer. It will cost the NHS ten times what it is worth - that's £1.2 billion.[16] It's the main reason why South London Healthcare Trust went bust in 2012. Norfolk and Norwich University Hospital is another PFI part-owned by Innisfree. A few years into the contract, the PFI owners refinanced it, raising their annual rate of return from 16 to 60 per cent.

There are many more Innisfree PFI timebombs detonating up and down the country - 19 in total. The healthcare of people in all these areas is jeopardised just so that chief executive David Metter and his total of 28 employees - yes that's right 28 - can make a killing![17] The *Daily Telegraph* describes him as 'the man, who owns 28 hospitals and a motorway'. At the last count, one might add.

Apparently there's no money left. Unless you are someone like **Metter, who took home £8.6 million in pay and dividends in 2010.**

Money that could have been used to treat patients, pay for more NHS staff and build more hospitals instead of cuts, sacking staff and closing hospitals. This is why Conservative MP Edward Leigh, chair of a Treasury Committee report on PFI, described it as the unacceptable face of capitalism.

The insidious encroachment of the private sector into the NHS had thus far been a salubrious warning of the unchartered waters that lay ahead. Or so you might have thought...

So the next time some minister or policy wonk bangs on about the NHS being unaffordable, it's worth remembering the scandalous cost of PFI. The toxic PFI debt has led to hospital mergers with consequent bed reductions, staff lay-offs and service closures. These mergers will be followed by the final 'wave of closures in the run-up to privatisation and franchising out'.[18] As Allyson Pollock astutely points out, the great irony is that PFI was once hailed as the largest hospital-building programme ever; in fact, it is the largest NHS hospital closure programme.

You bet there's an alternative

One begins to discern a pattern here. Could it be that those advocating bringing in the private sector do not have the interests of the NHS at heart? You would imagine that the case for terminating PFI, in the public interest, even if it means buying out or renegotiating the contracts, is a strong one. The National Audit Office recommended that the government should have the power to cancel contracts which are not providing value for money.[19] In fact, at least one hospital has done just that by buying out its PFI contract - West Park Hospital in Darlington (expected to save £14 million). However, this is not feasible for larger PFI contracts, such as Barts Health, without the backing of government.

The effective renationalisation of Network Rail and the London Underground Public-Private Partnership upgrade provide precedents.[20] However, this government does not have the political will to do this. They believe in the ideology of neoliberalism and are against the role of state provision.

In fact, the Treasury has been the midwife to PFI2 - a rebranding exercise, which sounds like a summer blockbuster sequel. Unfortunately it will be hospitals not movie villains which will be blown up as a result. It is likely that PFI2 - with higher rates of return for investors - will prove to be more expensive than the original PFI.[21]

Step Three: Facilitate the Corporate Takeover AKA Organise a Great Big Sell Off

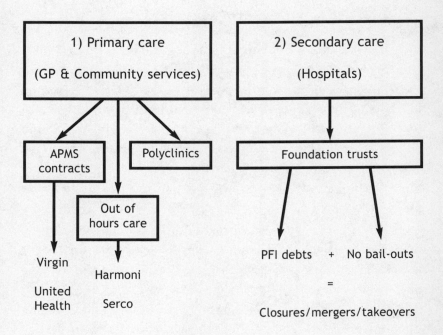

1) Primary care

The introduction of **Alternative Provider Medical Services (APMS)** contracts meant that Primary Care Trusts (PCTs) could commission care from companies employing salaried GPs rather than having traditional contracts with GPs themselves. Amongst the winners were UnitedHealth (more of whom later), Atos (to whom the government outsourced the controversial fitness tests for incapacity and other benefits) and Virgin.

The corporate takeover of **Out-of-Hours (OOH) Care** saw companies like Harmoni, Serco and Take Care Now win contracts to provide OOH care. Harmoni has been the leader in this field, quietly hoovering up whole swathes of OOH care nationwide.

2) Secondary care

Foundation trusts were introduced from 2003. This empty-sounding label essentially converted hospitals into semi-independent businesses with financial and other freedoms.

New GP and consultant contracts were negotiated in 2003-4. The GP contract appeared to be a major triumph. It made OOH care optional and led to increased pay for GP partners matching hospital consultant salaries. However, in the long run, it proved to be a significant own goal. Firstly, there was a backlash against GPs from Parliament, the CBI and the media, typified by the *Daily Mail*'s coruscating front pages slamming 'super GPs earning £250,000'. Never mind the distortion of this applying only to a tiny number of GPs, nor that the DoH had anticipated the majority of GPs opting out of OOH.[1]

Harmoni has been beset by allegations of cost-cutting, inadequate staffing and sub-standard care, most recently as part of *The Guardian*'s NHS Plc series. Serco and Take Care Now have also been implicated in similar controversies. **On at least one night, it is alleged that Serco had only one or two GPs covering most (if not all) of Cornwall. It was also claimed that Serco had falsified data to meet targets.**[2] A parliamentary report, by the Public Accounts Committee, highlighted this and accused the company of bullying employees. This contract has now been terminated. Serco has been dogged by scandals in recent times. *The Independent* revealed that Britain's largest pathology services provider, Viapath - established as a joint venture by Serco in partnership with Guy's and St Thomas' hospitals - has been **overcharging for diagnostic tests**. It is estimated that the amount could have been as high as £1 million in 2012 alone. There have also been safety concerns and pay cuts leading to loss of experienced staff.[3] If this all sounds familiar, that's because it is. Serco has been **under investigation by the Serious Fraud Office** for overcharging the government for electronic tagging of prisoners. Astonishingly, Serco continues to make profits from taxpayer money. 2013-14 NHS figures show that it was paid £10 million. G4S - also plagued by scandal - took £3.5 million.

None of this should surprise us as private companies only have one legal obligation, which is to their shareholders. In other words, their aim is to maximise profits usually through cutting staff and other costs. In this sense, the private sector can be seen to be more efficient.

The story behind these outfits is even more intriguing. *The Guardian* exposé describes how Harmoni was formed as a joint venture between the ECI private equity group and a GP co-operative.[4] Its annual turnover mushroomed from £3 million to £100 million. It was then sold to Care UK, which is owned by another private equity group - Bridgepoint - for £48 million. ECI took £20 million and the GP owners of the co-op became millionaires. We'll come back to the links between Care UK and the Tories later.

Virgin Assura claim to have a network of 30 GP partnerships with over 1500 GPs looking after 3 million patients. Astonishing figures when one is accustomed to thinking of the NHS as an impervious and timeless institution rather than one that is fragmenting as we speak. As of July 2010, 227 GP surgeries and health centres were privately run, with nine firms including Care UK holding ten or more contracts. Incidentally, the BMA (the doctors' union) negotiators set up a company by the name of Concordia Health and rapidly secured several APMS contracts.

What about the rest of primary care? In 2006-7, the government commissioned Lord Darzi to look into reconfiguring NHS services for the future. The brainchild of his report was the concept of a polyclinic. Polyclinics are large GP centres, with a wide variety of services that you might expect to find at a local hospital, including maternity care, mental health services, multidisciplinary teams, diagnostics and even specialist care. In fact, they seemed like such a good idea that they were rolled out nationwide, with the aim of having one polyclinic in every Primary Care Trust. There was just one snag. **Polyclinics, like everything else in this story, were inextricably linked to privatisation - they were on the whole to be privately financed and run.**

The running costs proved to be hideously expensive and, ultimately, their fate was ignominious. Although polyclinics were wound up, they have been the progenitors to a second wave of GP-led health centres based on APMS contracts. This rebranding was a misnomer obscuring their corporate nature.[5]

With general practice under this all-out assault, what of hospital care? From 2002 onwards, the DoH fixated on the model of **integrated care** utilised by Kaiser Permanente - a large California-based Health Maintenance Organisation (HMO), where the doctors are jointly partners and salaried employees. In a nutshell, integrated care is about the management of long-term conditions, through alternative systems and pathways to traditional methods (i.e. in hospital). This mainly involves managing these conditions in the community and keeping expensive, hospital care to a minimum. Again, not a bad idea in principle.

However, it is debatable as to whether integrated care is cheaper. Health economist Professor Maynard has cited many integrated care evaluations, including by the DoH, which demonstrate no savings.[6] In 2006, the NHS National Leadership Network produced a document stating that integrated care is not just about the shift of hospital care towards the community but the reconfiguration of NHS infrastructure. There would be a radical reduction in the number of NHS hospitals and the development of new facilities to house integrated care services 'decoupled' from the NHS. This would dovetail nicely with an expansion of the private sector. In other words, **there would be shrinkage of NHS-provided services with private ownership as the new norm.**

In fact, England has one of the lowest numbers of hospitals based on population, coming below Poland, Czech Republic, Estonia, Mexico and Korea.[7] It is important to bear this in mind when considering the current debate about closing down smaller hospitals and centralising services into large centres. This is purportedly justified on the basis that centralisation of services in large hospitals will deliver better care than in small cottage or district general hospitals.This may be sensible for highly specialised areas, such as trauma or stroke care. However, it is not necessarily best for common inpatient admissions (such as pneumonia), outpatient clinics and maternity care. In fact, most citizens are generally in favour of high quality local services for emergency, maternity, paediatric and elderly care.

Mental health was the testing ground for the integrated care plans being currently rolled out for physical health. The programme known as **Care in the Community** started in the 1980s under Thatcher resulting in the mass closure of NHS psychiatric hospitals, wards and beds. One of the results has been a drastic shortage of capacity for inpatient care. For example, children and adolescents are sometimes forced to travel hundreds of miles to access inpatient beds. Gradually, privatisation and outsourcing has been used to fill the gaps.

The Priory Group - long a byword for celebrity rehab - has become one of the main private providers of NHS mental health services. A total of 85 per cent of the Priory's income comes from the public sector. The NHS sends close to half of its child and adolescent inpatients to private hospitals. The Priory Group was sold for £1.3 billion by US private equity firm Advent International to Acadia Healthcare of Tennessee.

The shift towards community care also requires allocation of resources. In fact, the opposite has been happening with chronic under-investment in general practice. All in all, the evidence-base for these reconfigurations is shaky. It is likely that vested interests see service redesign as the pre-requisite for privatisation.

'Kaiser beacon' pilots have already been trialled and integrated care organisations have started springing up, such as Principia Partners in Health. Circle - the first private company to run an NHS hospital (Hinchingbrooke Hospital) - is very much based on the Kaiser model of co-ownership. However, this experiment has ended ignominiously with Circle's involvement deemed unsustainable and the hospital rated inadequate and put into special measures. **As a disclaimer, it should be mentioned that Kaiser are infamous for 'dumping' patients in downtown Los Angeles**. Yes, literally dumping patients in hospital gowns when their insurance policies have expired. There are over 50 such alleged cases. Not exactly the kind of ethos we should import over here.

When I was a junior doctor, I worked at Guy's and St Thomas' Hospital, which is a foundation trust, but I had no idea what this meant. Foundation trust status gave hospitals greater independence. For example, hospitals can make business partnerships. **The flip side is that foundation trusts are allowed to 'go bust'** as they are no longer eligible to be bailed out by the DoH. In this event, Monitor (the NHS regulator now part of NHS Improvement) can invite another trust to take over or alternatively leave the hospital to close. This was a paradigm shift as it forced hospitals to prioritise the bottom line over patient care.

A system of payment by results was also introduced, which meant hospitals being 'paid per completed treatment and not a lump sum for a given total'. These payments are based on 'a national tariff of fixed prices, adjusted for the seriousness of each category'.[8] Both foundation trusts and payment by results have increased administration and transaction costs. Transaction costs include: 'advertising, negotiating, contracting, invoicing, billing, auditing, monitoring contracts, collecting information, resolving disputes both in courts and out'.[9]

Many hospitals have rushed to attain foundation trust status. They have therefore needed to balance their books, which has often meant cutting frontline staff. **This was one of the main factors behind the Mid Staffs scandal, involving the deaths of hundreds of patients at Stafford Hospital in Staffordshire.** Poor care was not actually due to an uncaring ethos as has been suggested. It was often down to the lack of sufficient nursing staff on the wards as the Francis Inquiry concluded. In other words, this was yet another example of how market-based reforms have led to worse outcomes for the NHS and patients. Ironically, Mid Staffs then spent more on adequate staffing, went into deficit and was deemed unsustainable.

Foundation trust status may have seemed attractive but hospital bosses did not anticipate the current climate of cuts (including cuts to hospital tariffs) combined with mounting PFI debts. **As a result, tens of trusts up and down the country are running into the red. More than a third of acute NHS trusts in deficit are hospitals built under PFI.**[10]

Here are some of the corporate winners according to Colin Leys and Stewart Player in their book, *The Plot Against the NHS*:

- Private healthcare companies, both British, such as Care UK and Tribal, and international, such as Netcare (a South African hospital chain, which opened several ISTCs and bought a large chain of private hospitals) and UnitedHealth (commissioning contracts on behalf of CCGs)
- NHS IT contracts, e.g. the Connecting for Health (CfH) fiasco, NHS statistics, Dr Foster, NHS choices system (previously run by Capita)
- Big Seven companies in hospital cleaning, catering, laundry (with annual revenues totalling £2 billion)
- PFI consortia (£7.1 billion estimated revenue from 2010/11-2015/16 - corresponding to almost half the savings the NHS was forced to make in the same period)

So who really are the beneficiaries of this hidden hand? The scale of the 'marketiser's network', as labelled by corporate watchdog Spinwatch, is vast. Let's start with Serco - a *Guardian* profile described it as 'the biggest company you've never heard of':

> As well as five British prisons and the tags attached to over 8,000 English and Welsh offenders, Serco sees to two immigration removal centres...You'll also see its logo on the Docklands Light Railway and Woolwich ferry, and it is a partner in both Liverpool's Merseyrail network, and the Northern Rail franchise...Serco runs school inspections in parts of England, speed cameras all over the UK, and the National Nuclear Laboratory, based at the Sellafield site in Cumbria. It also holds the contracts for the management of the UK's ballistic missile early warning system on the Yorkshire moors...But even this is only a fraction of the story. Among their scores of roles across the planet, Serco is responsible for air traffic control in the United Arab Emirates, parking-meter services in Chicago, driving tests in Ontario, and an immigration detention centre on Christmas Island.[11]

The *Daily Telegraph* puts it bluntly: 'Without Serco, Britain would struggle to go to war.' The parallels with a *New York Times* profile of Lockheed Martin (potentially bidding for NHS contracts) are clear to see:

> Lockheed Martin doesn't run the United States. But it does help run a breathtakingly big part of it. Over the last decade, Lockheed, the nation's largest military contractor, has built a formidable information-technology empire that now stretches from the Pentagon to the post office. It sorts your mail and totals your taxes. It cuts Social Security checks and counts the United States census. It runs space flights and monitors air traffic. To make all that happen, Lockheed writes more

computer code than Microsoft.[12]

The South African company **Netcare** is one of the leading lights in private hospital chains. Netcare has been implicated in illegal kidney transplants with the knowledge of its chief executive, according to South African prosecutors. Although it has denied some of these allegations, it has admitted to receiving £342,000 from an organ trafficking syndicate for assisting with **illegal kidney transplants including from five children**.[13]

Next up is UnitedHealth Group, the single largest health carrier in the US and one of the top ten Fortune 500 US corporations with an annual revenue of $120 billion in 2014.[14] Remarkably, UnitedHealth's annual revenue soared to $200 billion in 2017. In 2009, their CEO pocketed over $100 million (I would have to work for 1700 years to earn this sum!). **UnitedHealth** have been repeatedly forced to pay massive fines for **multiple instances of fraud** involving various branches of the US government. The share options scam involving the DoH's Channing Wheeler and previous CEO Dr William McGuire led to UnitedHealth being forced to hand back hundreds of millions of dollars to shareholders. **The State of California was seeking nearly $10 billion in fines**, although this has been revised significantly downwards.[15] UnitedHealth has also been the subject of a class action lawsuit filed by the American Medical Association claiming that it used faulty claims data to underpay doctors and overcharge patients. The New York Attorney General said patients had been victims of 'consumer fraud' for a decade in a settlement that saw UnitedHealth pay $350 million in compensation. The updated company database has more recently been generating controversy for using algorithms to calculate the most expensive patients and the doctors with the fewest patients. For companies like UnitedHealth, these fines are loose pocket change. This is just part and parcel of how they do business.

Dr William McGuire's exit compensation is said to have been - wait for it - $1.1 billion. In the US, healthcare-related fraud is endemic. UnitedHealth has run GP surgeries and is one of the major players in commissioning. UnitedHealth has also paid for senior NHS executives to travel to the US to see how the company operates and explore applicability in the UK. It is remarkable that we are opening the door in Britain to these multinationals mired in scandal and fraud. Perhaps this is what Jeremy Hunt means by rediscovering a caring ethos in the NHS. Remember that NHS England chief executive Simon Stevens used to work for UnitedHealth, so yet again we shouldn't be too surprised.[16]

And then there is **McKinsey**. The US firm is the largest management consultancy in the world. The *Mail on Sunday* described it as the firm that hijacked the NHS in an exposé revealing how it had lavished NHS regulators, drawn up proposals for the HSCA and used access to share information with other clients.[17]

McKinsey's fingerprints are all over NHS reforms. We have already come across Penny Dash, behind the NHS Plan 2000 and the Darzi plans for polyclinics, and Dr David Bennett, former McKinsey director and former chief executive of Monitor. McKinsey produced the 2008 report NHS London and the 2009 financial analysis behind the efficiency savings (cuts of £15-20 billion up to 2015). The efficiency savings have been extended to 2020 thus amounting to around £40 billion over this decade.

In a climate of economic stagnation, corporations are turning to opening the oyster of European public services in order to continue generating massive profits. The NHS alone represents over a staggering £120 billion per year.

Step Four: Install a Revolving Door

How did all of this happen? The short answer is the **revolving door**. Former secretaries of state for health and health ministers (such as Lord Warner) packed their bags after discharging their public duties and headed for the lucrative pastures of post-Westminster retirement in the private sector.

After his departure as health secretary, Andrew Lansley went on to advise pharmaceutical giant Roche, private equity leviathan Blackstone, management consultants Bain & Company and UKActive (sponsored by Coca Cola amongst others).[1]

As Colin Leys and Stewart Player have pointed out, **Alan Milburn** (Secretary of State for Health 1999-2003) went on to become an adviser to Bridgepoint Capital (a private equity firm involved in financing Alliance Medical and Care UK), Lloyds Pharmacy, Covidien (medical suppliers) and Pepsico. **Patricia Hewitt** was Secretary of State for Health 2005-7. Hewitt then became adviser to private equity company Cinven (which bought Bupa's chain of 25 private hospitals) and was paid £60,000 for 18 days' work a year. She was also a 'special consultant' to Alliance Boots at an annual salary of £40,000 and a non-executive director of BT at a salary of £60,000. In the cash for access scandal, she was caught by Channel 4's *Dispatches* offering to use her contacts 'on behalf of the imaginary clients of a fictitious US lobbying firm for £3,000 a day'.

Further down the pyramid, Alan Milburn's team consisted of Simon Stevens, private secretary Tony Sampson and media adviser Andrew Harrison. **Stevens,** Blair's senior health policy adviser, went to work for UnitedHealth (as an executive vice president) and eventually came back to haunt us (through said revolving door) as no less than the chief executive of NHS England.

Stevens was not the only one to go on to work with

UnitedHealth. Sampson was UnitedHealth's chief lobbyist in the UK between 2005 and 2013, whilst Harrison is head of health at lobbying firm Hanover, which has lobbied for UnitedHealth since 2007. The former *BMJ* editor Richard Smith also went to work for UnitedHealth.[2]

As early as 2003, UnitedHealth was providing administrative health services to ten Primary Care Trusts and Kaiser Permanente was engaged with eight PCTs. The intention of the New Labour government was to develop integrated care models. Alan Milburn asked DoH officials 'to enter into discussions to explore the potential for and feasibility of adapting and applying United Healthcare's Evercare model in a number of PCTs'.[3]

Yet who really is Simon Stevens? Mention his name to most NHS staff and you will draw a blank. This anonymity certainly works in his favour once you probe deeper. His track record at UnitedHealth speaks for itself. He lobbied against Obamacare, which only entailed moderate reforms and nothing like the universal healthcare system that is so badly needed in the US. In fact, the US health insurance sector lobbied intensively, including astro-turfing (creating fake grassroots campaigns), in order to neutralise a public option that would have competed with private insurance plans.

Stevens lobbied for the Transatlantic Trade and Investment Partnership (TTIP) - the EU-US trade agreement. TTIP threatens to open up European public services for corporate takeover. It could then lock in this privatisation by potentially handing corporations the right to sue governments if their policies harm profits or even the future expectation of profits. More than half of the world's countries have already been sued by investors as a result of other similar trade agreements. Thus TTIP would have further opened up the NHS to privatisation and acted as a deterrent to any government trying to restore the NHS as a public healthcare system. Stevens also lobbied for the global expansion of UnitedHealth into Europe, India and China.

As head of the European division of UnitedHealth, Stevens was key to them winning the right to take over two GP practices in Derbyshire (since sold). Stevens co-authored a report for UnitedHealth arguing that the Obama administration could save $500 billion in Medicare and Medicaid funding over 10 years by aggressively coordinating medical care for pensioners and the poor.

Stevens was also a founder member of healthcare lobbying coalition The Alliance for Healthcare Competitiveness (AHC). AHC wants the US government to build its free trade policy around the healthcare industry by breaking down tariffs in order to export its 'health ecosystem' internationally. According to OpenDemocracy, AHC is in favour of less regulation of drug quality and price and a ban on favouring state providers like the NHS over private companies.[4]

Stevens reportedly stated that ageing populations worldwide will lead to a demand for goods and services that can drive sales of American insurance, medical devices and record-keeping technology. Stevens was also reported as stating that UnitedHealth is negotiating to provide a private health insurance programme in India that could include one million people.[5]

It was therefore surprising that *The Guardian*'s health correspondent, Denis Campbell, hailed the return of Stevens with a puff piece in which the headline read 'Simon Stevens' switch to NHS is "like Arsenal signing Mesut Ozil"'. The Ozil comparison came unsurprisingly from health lobbyist Mike Birtwistle at Incisive Health. The article began by noting that the appointment prompted 'widespread relief, a broad consensus that he is the right choice'. However the profile did note that Stevens had been instrumental in the setting up of ISTCs, foundation trusts and that he is an advocate of local pay. [6] Similarly, Evan Davis kicked off a debate on BBC *Newsnight* with the same sentiment that this was the best man for the job. *The Independent* was somewhat more sceptical of Stevens' appointment asking whether he really was the right person to run the NHS.[7]

So what does Simon say? Speaking to *The Independent* in 2015, Stevens stated that the NHS has no choice but to change the way it provides care through radical reforms (towards a US model of care known as accountable or integrated care) moving care away from hospitals otherwise it would become unaffordable.[8] Stevens has stated that he secured an extra £8 billion for the NHS budget by 2020. What he forgot to mention is £22 billion more in cuts to meet the funding gap of £30 billion. Stevens also states that the NHS needs devolution with regional control of health and social care budgets. This will mean devolving cuts in a time of austerity. This pooling of budgets will see the NHS competing against local authorities for scarce funds. It will mean denationalisation with the erosion of national standards for patients and staff resulting in an even more fragmented, regional service. It will also mean the merging of health and social care budgets with healthcare becoming increasingly privatised and means-tested just like social care.

The revolving door turns smoothly in both directions. Management consultants from McKinsey, KPMG, Deloitte and Atos, to name a few, infiltrated the top tiers of the DoH. A similar pattern emerges across NHS management. This is how the health policy community was hijacked.

NHS England's deputy chief executive, Ian Dalton, left for BT in February 2013. Whilst Dalton ran their 'global health division, BT received £18 million in contracts from NHS England'.[9] Former Monitor chief executive David Bennett 'spent 18 years with McKinsey before becoming chief policy adviser to Tony Blair and head of the Prime Minister's Strategy Unit'. We'll come back to other links between Monitor and McKinsey. Penny Dash was head of strategy at the DoH before joining McKinsey. Whilst there, she developed the NHS Plan 2000, which expanded the internal market. She also co-founded the Cambridge Health Network, which aims to bring NHS and private healthcare leaders together. Tom Kibasi rejoined McKinsey after 2 years out as senior policy adviser to former NHS chief executive David Nicholson. He is now the director of the Institute for Public Policy Research (IPPR) think-tank. [10]

In 2009, it was estimated that spending on management consultants alone was upwards of £300 million a year.[11] Andrew Lansley, former Conservative health secretary, stated that he was 'staggered by the scale of the expenditure'. However, since the Coalition came to power, management consultant fees have doubled to £640 million.[12] It seems that austerity, like taxes, only applies to the little people.

The results of this management consultancy culture have included PFIs and CfH. The latter is the **national NHS IT programme - recommended by McKinsey and run by a consultant from Deloitte - which is largely non-operational at a haemorrhaging cost of £20 billion**. This is equivalent to the entire efficiency savings (based on a set of 120 PowerPoint slides prepared by McKinsey) the NHS was asked to make between 2011 and 2014.

However, some of these costs could have been mitigated. Richard Granger (Director-General of the NHS National Programme for IT) did not charge Accenture £1 billion as permitted by the contract when they withdrew from the project in 2006. Instead they were only fined £63 million. Granger's next job was with Andersen Consulting (later Accenture).[13]

The revolving door spins into Downing Street. **Nick Seddon** was David Cameron's health adviser. Here are OpenDemocracy and Social Investigations on his background:

Seddon's last role was as deputy director of 'Reform' - a free market think-tank extensively funded by healthcare and insurance companies. **He has openly called for an end to the NHS as we know it, and promoted the idea of an insurance-based system**...A *Telegraph* article by Seddon highlighted a Reform report, titled 'It can be done', which praised the increased involvement of private companies in running hospitals in Spain and Germany.

No prizes for guessing why Seddon is in favour of all this. He was previously head of communications at Circle, which you will recall became the first private company to run an NHS hospital at Hinchingbrooke.

This is what he had to say on CCGs: 'There is no evidence to suggest that they [GPs] have the skills needed, which makes it unlikely that they'll be any good at trying to make hospitals improve what they do and cut their costs...'

However, CCGs could be used as the basis to move towards a 'mixed funding insurance model. **The £80 billion budget could be allocated to insurers in professional alliances with GP groups...those who can afford to would be encouraged to contribute more towards their care packages.**'[14]

This kind of remark is very useful. Every now and again, there is an unguarded comment from those in the know, devoid of all spin. Seddon is clearly referring to healthcare insurance. And this is exactly how we should view CCGs - as insurance pools. The concept of a National Health Service has been replaced by insurance pools allocating the central government funding stream (increasingly to private companies) with tighter criteria leading to greater rationing of treatment. Seddon has gone on to work as an executive for the UK arm of UnitedHealth - Optum.

Over 200 parliamentarians have recent past or present financial interests in companies involved in private healthcare - 147 Lords and 73 MPs - according to Social Investigations. *The Mirror* listed 70 MPs with links to private healthcare.[15] No surprise then that they are selling off our NHS.

Private companies with financial links to Conservative politicians have won contracts worth £1.5 billion, according to research by the largest trade union, Unite. The most notorious example of this is the former health secretary and architect of the reforms, Lord Andrew Lansley, receiving a donation of £21,000 from Caroline Nash, the wife of John Nash. At the time, John Nash was the chairman of private healthcare company Care UK.[16]

The notion of a boundary between the public and private sectors, which should be policed in the public interest, has long been expunged. There is certainly something rotten in the state of the NHS but, contrary to what the right-wing media and the Conservatives espouse, it is most definitely not NHS care or staff. And when the stench is so overwhelming then you have to call it what it is - Corruption with a capital C; the kind of corruption normally associated with mafia states and banana republics.

Step Five: Run a PR Smear Campaign

The relentless anti-NHS smear campaign, run by various sectors of the media, is now escalating, softening up the public in preparation for the expansion of private health insurance coverage. Certainly the proliferation of private healthcare ads suggests that insurance companies are already licking their lips at this mouthwatering prospect. There is a simple test to establish whether this is indeed a PR campaign. Who runs the NHS? The government of course, stupid. And yet there has been not so much as a murmur of protest in defence of this all-out assault on *its* NHS.

There has been neither a democratic mandate nor an evidence-base for these reforms. Factsheets on the DoH website summarise the government's case for change.[1] This is largely premised upon affordability (notably in the context of the current state of the nation's finances) and modernising the NHS to improve standards. If you believe what you read in the papers then these arguments would seem utterly persuasive. There have been consistent doubts cast, in the media, on the affordability of the NHS and on the standard of care it provides. This aids the government's agenda of promoting reform but the real data undermines this case.

Is the NHS Affordable?
This is one of the key questions. I repeatedly hear colleagues and friends ask, 'But where will the money come from?'

John Appleby, the Chief Economist at the King's Fund, has largely dismantled the case that the NHS is unaffordable in the pages of the *BMJ*.[2] We'll let the charts do the talking...

Here are the Organisation for Economic Co-operation and Development (OECD) figures in health spending:

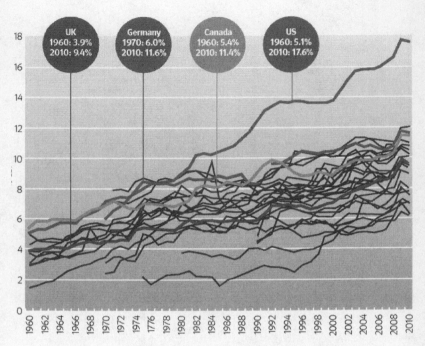

Approaching £1 in £10 of its economic wealth, in 2010 the UK devoted more than twice the share of gross domestic product (GDP) to public plus private healthcare spending as it did in 1960. The US spent around 5 per cent of GDP on healthcare in 1960. Today it is nudging 18 per cent, and in total the US spends almost the same on health as all other countries in the OECD put together. Germany, France and the Netherlands now spend around €1 in €8 on healthcare.

Reproduced with permission of the author John Appleby from 'Rises in healthcare spending: where will it end?' Published in the *BMJ* in 2012.[refers to Figure 3]

Here are the figures for EU-15 countries health spending:

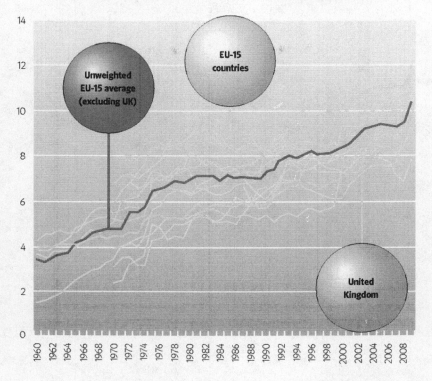

Total healthcare spending of EU-15 countries (Austria, Belgium, Denmark, Finland, France, Germany, Greece, Ireland, Italy, Luxembourg, the Netherlands, Portugal, Spain, Sweden and UK) as a proportion of GDP, 1960-2008. Unweighted average=sum of percentages/number of countries submitting data in each year.

Reproduced with permission of the author John Appleby from 'Can we afford the NHS in future?' Published 12/7/11 *BMJ* 2011;343:d4321 [refers to Figure 4]

In a 2011 paper, John Appleby cites an article Andrew Lansley wrote in the *Telegraph*, in which he stated that by 2030, 'If things carry on unchanged, this would mean real terms health spending more than doubling to £230 billion' and that 'this is something we simply cannot afford'.[3]

Healthcare spending is at around 7 per cent of GDP. As Appleby surmises, based on projections, £230 billion as a proportion of GDP in 2030 will amount to 10.9 per cent. 'Adding private spending on healthcare to NHS spend (to enable better comparison with other countries), total spend in 2030 could be around 12.4% of GDP.'

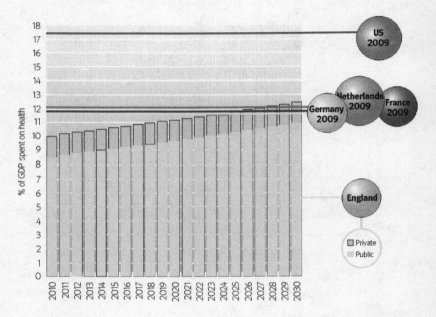

Possible future English healthcare spending 2010-30 as proportion of GDP. Figures are hypothetical and assume English private spending is 1.5 per cent of GDP.

Reproduced with permission of the author John Appleby from 'Can we afford the NHS in future?' Published 12/7/11 *BMJ* 2011;343:d4321

As Appleby concludes, 'this would make England the highest spending country in the OECD bar the US - but only assuming no other country increased its spending on healthcare. Even in 2009, seven of the EU-15 countries spent over 10% of GDP on healthcare. The highest spender - the Netherlands - devoted 12%

of its GDP to healthcare.'

In fact, UK spending on healthcare is less than all other G7 countries apart from Italy, which spends the same, according to the Office for National Statistics (ONS). On current projections, UK spending could even fall to 6 per cent of GDP by 2021 (due to cuts) according to the King's Fund think-tank.[4]

In summary, there are two key points. First, rising healthcare costs are a fact across the world.[5] Second, **the NHS is one of the most inexpensive healthcare systems** in the developed world. We have already seen how market-based reforms - such as the internal market, foundation trusts and payment by results - actually increase costs. Bringing in the private sector - in the form of PFIs or ISTCs to name two examples - has generally lined the pockets of corporations whilst producing worse outcomes for the NHS and patients, not to mention running hospitals into the ground.

Market-based healthcare systems tend to be more expensive than the NHS. In the 1960s, the economist and Nobel laureate Kenneth Arrow demonstrated that the normal rules of the market do not apply to healthcare. The US system is the best example of this, with healthcare costs going through the roof. This is because classical market forces do not exert the usual control and do not regulate supply and demand. Physicians are paid through a fee-for-service system, which basically means that the more they do, the more they are paid. Likewise, hospitals and laboratories aim to increase their services to maximise profits. Pharmaceuticals and medical manufacturers also promote their products aggressively. Combine all of this with minimal regulation of prices, add in for-profit private insurance plans with some giant insurance corporations, and you have a system in which costs are out of control, driven by profit incentives and not by medical need. Unsurprisingly, this set-up encourages gaming of the system with fraudulent billing and inflated charges accounting for a significant amount of healthcare fraud.[6]

The question should not be whether we can afford the NHS but what kind of healthcare system do we want?

An NHS England document - 'The NHS belongs to the people' - projects a £30 billion funding gap by 2020.[7] Hence Professor Malcolm Grant, NHS England chairman, airing that **post-2015 NHS user charges would need to be considered**. This is the man who has been on record as saying, 'I don't use the NHS.'[8] Migrant charges have been brought in, introducing a charging mechanism into the NHS. Meanwhile, the bilious tabloids foment about health tourism - accounting for 0.3 per cent of the budget and distracting from over £300 billion of UK PFI debt being siphoned to corporates and banks.

However, there is a simple reason why we do not generally have user charges. Successive governments have undertaken major reviews of NHS funding, including Sir Derek Wanless' 2002 report for the Treasury. They have all concluded that central taxation is the most efficient and fairest system.[9] Before the efficiency savings started to bite, ministers handed back a £2.2 billion underspend from the NHS budget to the Treasury in 2013 following an underspend of over £1.4 billion similarly handed back in 2012.[10]

The Nuffield Trust think-tank produced a paper - 'A Decade of Austerity?' - projecting that the efficiency savings should be extended.[11] The question appears to have been rhetorical. Efficiency savings have now been extended until 2021 and **could even reach £50 billion** by 2019-20, according to the DoH.[12,13]

On international comparisons, NHS performance is good. **The US-based Commonwealth Fund's large study of 20,000 patients in 11 industrialised countries found the NHS to be almost the least costly and to have almost the best levels of access.**

Other countries not only spent more per head but also charged patients directly, reducing equality of access. Only

Switzerland reported faster access to care but Switzerland also spent some 35 per cent more per head than the UK. Only New Zealand spent less per head but one in seven said they skipped hospital visits because of cost. In the US, which spent almost twice as much per head as the UK, one in three Americans avoided seeking care because of cost.[14]

This report was updated in 2014 and 2017 by the Commonwealth Fund finding that, **'The United Kingdom ranks first overall, scoring highest on quality, access and efficiency.'**[15] But you will not have seen this headline carried by many newspapers: NHS BEST HEALTH SYSTEM IN THE WORLD! On the other hand, the US was castigated as the worst of the 11 countries despite putting the most money into health.[16]

The OECD's *Health at a Glance* (2011), one of the most respected sources of international comparisons, corroborated this picture of the NHS being amongst the best in the world. According to their head of health, Mark Pearson, 'The UK is one of the best performers in the world.' The DoH grudgingly conceded that the NHS is performing well for patients. The OECD also emphasised that the NHS has cut heart attack deaths by two-thirds since 1980. Less than 5 per cent of adults had diabetes in 2010, contrasting with 10 per cent in the US.[17]

This is not to say that the NHS does not have weaknesses. As with any system in the world, there is room for improvement, including mortality rates in certain types of cancer. There are also more avoidable hospital admissions for asthma in the UK than the average in the OECD.

Admittedly, there has been a deterioration in performance indicators more recently but this is somewhat attributable to a manufactured crisis created by deliberate policies.

In recent years, there have been a number of scandals involving hospital care. Whilst the media are very good at exposing NHS deficiencies, there is only glib analysis of the factors behind this.

The Guardian managed to run a double page story on the financial troubles of Barts Health, with PFI mentioned as an afterthought.[18] You may recall that we are talking about a £6 billion funding gap generated by its PFI. Quite an omission! Hospitals are operating in a climate of stealth cuts and massive PFI debts leading to them cutting frontline staff and diverting money away from patient care. As a result, delivery of care has been compromised. These stories present the NHS in a bad light without any explanation.

Take the A&E crisis splashed across the front pages every winter. The take-home message seems to be that the NHS is creaking at the seams and can no longer take the strain. The reality behind the A&E crisis is that it has largely been manufactured due to long-standing problems. For starters, 40 per cent of walk-in centres have been closed since 2010.[19] This is compounded by **a reduction in bed numbers of over 50 per cent since 1987-8** - from nearly 300,000 down to just 135,000.[20] Britain now has one of the lowest numbers of beds in all of Europe. In fact, hospitals are spending millions buying up increased bed capacity at private hospital chains run by the likes of BMI and Spire.[21] The same companies are bidding for NHS work and are often owned by large private equity firms. This is a case of NHS budgets being simultaneously squeezed on more than one front.

At the same time, there has been a steep decline in the provision of social care whilst the elderly population and demand have both increased. This means that elderly patients cannot be discharged safely and they end up 'bed-blocking', which therefore has a knock-on effect. In October 2017, there were a total of over 170,000 bed days - when a patient stays in a hospital bed overnight - taken up by patients fit to leave but who could not be discharged due to lack of social care support. In August 2010, there were just 55,332 bed days lost.[22] This is certainly a scenario familiar to every junior doctor.

But the problem is getting worse as local councils tighten eligibility criteria due to massive austerity cuts. **The number of**

elderly and disabled people receiving care at home has been slashed by a third in the past few years.[23] These patients are thus more likely to end up in A&E. In fact, you cannot separate out the A&E crisis from the historic social care crisis. Long-term residential care was privatised from Thatcher onwards and by the end of the 1990s, free long-term care provided by the NHS had largely been replaced by private sector care homes charging fees.[24]

In view of all of this, it's not exactly surprising that A&Es are struggling to cope.

John Appleby has examined some of the trends in NHS performance in a paper entitled 'Does poor health justify NHS reform?' The official ministerial briefing for the Health & Social Care Bill stated the rate of death from heart disease is double that of France. Age standardised death rate for heart attacks was around 19/100,000 in France and 41/100,000 in the UK. But this is only true comparing just one year (2006) with the country with the lowest death rate for heart attacks in Europe. The UK has had lower levels of spending every year for the past half century than France. OECD spending comparisons show that in 2008, the UK spent 8.7 per cent of its GDP on health compared with 11.2 per cent for France.[25]

The bigger picture is that the UK has experienced the largest fall in deaths from heart attacks, between 1980 and 2006, of any European country.

Jeremy Hunt himself penned an article in *The Guardian* celebrating that 'patients who have heart surgery in England have a greater chance of survival than in almost any other European country. Since 2005, death rates have halved and are now far lower than the European average.'[26] Why? Because the surgeons decided to collect, analyse and publish their own data with openness leading to greater success. In other words, improvements in the NHS or any public sector organisation can be achieved without recourse to marketisation or privatisation.

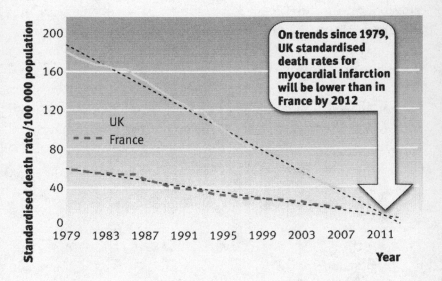

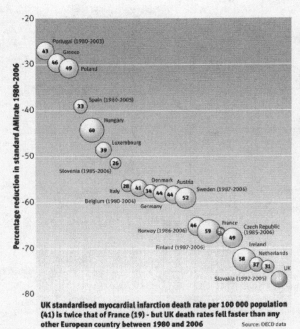

Reproduced with permission of the author John Appleby from 'Does poor health justify NHS reform?' Published 28/1/11 *BMJ* 2011;342:d566

In the same paper, Appleby goes on to examine cancer data. In the UK, death rates for **lung cancer** in men rose to a peak in 1979. Since then they have steadily fallen and are now **lower than for French men**. With regards to **breast cancer** mortality - 'since 1989, age standardised death rates per 100,000 in the UK have fallen by 40% to virtually close the gap with France, where they have fallen by just 10%...if trends continue, **it is likely that the UK will have lower death rates than France in just a few years'**.

The Eurocare study - the most comprehensive ongoing study of cancer survival across Europe - often feeds headlines that the UK is the 'sick man of Europe'. Trends from Eurocare actually show improvements in survival rates for the UK - confirmed by the Office for National Statistics (ONS). But Eurocare is problematic, with a lag in data several years behind, and patchy coverage (French data cover around 10-15 per cent of people with cancer, whilst UK data cover 100 per cent).

It is also worth bearing in mind that whether one is looking at heart disease or cancer, there are extrinsic factors (such as changing lifestyle patterns or public awareness) not directly connected to the performance of a healthcare system.

And what of the public? As Nicholas Timmins points out, **public satisfaction with the NHS was at its highest ever (as recorded by the British Social Attitudes Survey)** just as the white paper for the Health & Social Care Bill was launched. This is a polling series stretching back to 1983.[27] DoH patient surveys were showing the same thing. **Polling in 2012 showed the NHS to be more popular than even the monarchy.**[28]

We can see that affordability, standards and public satisfaction far from justify a massive upheaval of the NHS. Not only is the cost of the Coalition's reconfiguration estimated at up to £3 billion but the OECD has stated that such endless reforms are actually holding back the NHS. Mark Pearson, head of health at the OECD, points out that 'each reform costs two years of improvements in quality. No country reforms its health service as frequently as the UK.'[29]

Many of the myths and misconceptions surrounding the NHS are often perpetuated by those with a hidden agenda or a vested interest in undermining the NHS. The simple truth is that key establishment figures in the government and media cannot stand the idea of a National Health Service and its public provision of healthcare free at the point of delivery. It is an affront to everything they espouse - that the public sector is inefficient and bureaucratic, that privatisation and markets are always good and that state provision is to be limited as much as possible.

Step Six. Legislate for the Dismantling of the NHS

Just as I was signing off our panel's report on 'Delivering real choice' I get sent a copy of the PM's speech announcing he was accepting many of our key recommendations (although we haven't actually given him the report yet!)...

Sir Stephen Bubb, who reviewed the role of competition in the NHS for the Health & Social Care Bill.[1]

Tony Benn once predicted a revolution in the streets if the NHS was privatised. On the opposite benches, Nigel Lawson, Thatcher's former chancellor, acknowledged that the NHS is 'the closest thing the English have to a religion'. Therefore the Conservatives knew they could not touch the NHS in the public glare. This had to be undertaken by stealth. Nicholas Timmins has diligently charted this process in *Never Again: The Story of the Health & Social Care Act*.[2] Labour's mantra 'you can't trust the Tories with the NHS' has resonated for many years with the British public. After David Cameron became party leader in 2005, the Tories pulled out all the stops in order to detoxify how they were perceived on the NHS. Cameron, a former Carlton man, knows a thing or two about PR. This was in keeping with the rebranding of the Conservatives as compassionate, repositioning the party towards the centre-ground. The message was 'the NHS is safe in our hands'. The 2010 manifesto promised: 'We are stopping the top-down reconfigurations of NHS services, imposed from Whitehall.'

Only weeks into government, the Tories reverted to form. The mother of all reconfigurations was unveiled in the white paper 'Liberating the NHS' and all hell broke loose.[3] David Nicholson, the NHS chief executive at the time, remarked that the change was so large it was visible from space.[4] The Health & Social Care

Bill met with fierce opposition from every conceivable quarter forcing the government to pause for a 'listening exercise'. However, according to *The Guardian* and *Social Investigations*, **a leaked document revealed that 'the private health lobby worked with Downing Street behind the scenes to ensure that the new legislation went ahead'.**[5]

David Worskett, one of the main lobbyists for the private healthcare industry, wrote in a memo at the time: 'the whole sequence of *Telegraph* articles and editorials on the importance of the Government not going soft on public service reform, including some strong pieces on health, is something I have been orchestrating and working with Reform to bring about'.[6]

The Coalition then embarked on a charm offensive. Cabinet members were wheeled out one after another to placate us with homilies. Not least of all Andrew Lansley, reasserting time and again how passionate he is about the NHS and how cherished it is as a British institution. For the above, read as eulogies. In the words of the doctor and *Daily Telegraph* columnist Max Pemberton, the death warrant had been issued.[7] You know the writing is on the wall when this much praise is being heaped on the NHS by the party who voted against its establishment and have fought against it ever since. As James Meek put it in the *London Review of Books,* you can praise something whilst at the same time legislating it out of existence.[8]

The political capital expended has been massive, with public opinion turning against the government handling of the NHS. It is all in keeping with the Coalition's growing reputation for *omnishambles*. However, don't let that fool you. An intriguing question is why the Tories chose to execute this so soon after the election campaign despite repeated avowals to the contrary. The answer may lie in Tony Blair's purported advice to them, which was paraphrased as ramming the Bill through as swiftly as possible because the public will have forgotten about it by the time of the next election.[9]

The Coalition emphasised the motifs of the Bill as improving patient choice through competition, empowering doctors and cutting management costs, neatly encapsulated in the euphemistic title of the white paper as 'Liberating the NHS' - all of which is nothing less than a smokescreen for the implementation of free market reforms. The Health & Social Care document weighs in at a door-stopping 473 pages (tellingly over four times the size of the original 1948 legislation that set up the NHS). But there are only three words that really matter - **ANY QUALIFIED PROVIDER**. This should really serve as the epitaph on the Coalition government's obituary. It means that **tendering of NHS contracts will be opened up to providers from the voluntary and more importantly private sectors**.

Professor Martin McKee, Professor of European Public Health at the London School of Hygiene and Tropical Medicine, dubbed the Act's sheer length and complexity as the Jackson Pollock effect. The Act is said to have been drawn up by a group of corporate lawyers. Professor McKee also compares it to the Schleswig-Holstein question - an arcane complex of diplomatic issues arising in the nineteenth century relating to the two eponymous duchies. British Prime Minister Lord Palmerston is reported to have said at the time, 'Only three people...have ever really understood the Schleswig-Holstein business - the Prince Consort, who is dead - a German professor, who has gone mad - and I, who have forgotten all about it.'

In other words, the Bill amounted to deliberate obfuscation that left critics floundering whilst the government got on with the real business of carving up the NHS. Don't take my word for it. Those are the words of Mark Britnell, an NHS manager who became one of the most powerful civil servants in the DoH.

As James Meek has assiduously documented, Britnell went on to work as global head of health for the consultants KPMG...In 2010 Britnell was interviewed for...a conference in New York: 'In future,' Britnell said, 'the NHS will be a state insurance provider, not a state deliverer…The NHS will be shown no mercy and the best time to take advantage of this will be in the next couple of years.'[10]

The Britnell quote is shocking enough but this was no ordinary conference. Its subject was

'how private companies could take advantage of the vulnerability of healthcare systems in a harsh financial climate'.[11]

This is another of these unguarded and illuminating quotes. The NHS is basically being converted into a state insurance provider similar to Medicare and Medicaid in the US with CCGs, based on US-managed care organisations, acting as healthcare insurers.

That Britnell was a serious candidate for the most important position in the NHS - the chief executive designate of the NHS Commissioning Board - is a damning indictment and helps explain how we got into this mess in the first place. The position eventually went to the incumbent NHS chief executive David Nicholson, who fawningly described the reforms as 'really, really revolutionary'.[12] Britnell has since told the *BMJ* that he is keen to come back to the NHS.

So what does the Act do? According to the BMA:

- The Act places duties on the Secretary of State for Health to promote a comprehensive health service in England.
- The Act enables the Secretary of State to set priorities for the NHS through a mandate for the NHS Commissioning Board.
- The Act also establishes CCGs to be responsible for commissioning local services.[13]

All of this sounds perfectly anodyne until you decipher the legalese. This is what Allyson Pollock, David Price and Peter Roderick have done in the *BMJ*. Firstly, the Act severs the duty of the health secretary to provide a national health service by devolving this to CCGs. CCGs, unlike PCTs, will not have to provide health services for everyone living in their area but only those on the patient lists of GPs. This is an important distinction and allows **exclusion of patients**. There are other exclusionary criteria. CCGs can also decide on what services will be free at the point of delivery. The legislation states that they have the power to determine what is **'appropriate as part of the health service'**. Vague indeed. In other words, the Act undermines the legal requirement for CCGs to provide comprehensive care. This means that there will be increased rationing, which fits in with the concept of CCGs as insurance pools with the potential to exclude some patients from coverage.

The authors conclude that:

> **The Act legislates for 'reductions in government funded health services as a consequence of decisions made independently of the secretary of state by a range of bodies... [It fails] to make clear who is ultimately responsible for people's health services...creates new powers for charging [and]...signals the basis for a shift from a mainly tax financed health service to one in which patients may have to pay for services currently free at point of delivery'.**[14]

Monitor (now part of NHS Improvement) will be the economic regulator for all NHS-funded services. It has many roles, including the prevention of anti-competitive behaviour. According to the BMA, 'Monitor will also have powers to assist providers in significant difficulty. This will include requiring a provider to appoint a turnaround expert to help them avoid failure and appointing a continuity administrator to take control of a provider's affairs when it is deemed clinically or financially unsustainable.'

Now let's take a closer look at former and present members

on the **board** of Monitor:[15]

- Dr David Bennett (former chief executive of Monitor), ex senior partner at McKinsey & Co (18 years).
- Keith Palmer (former deputy chairman of Monitor), ex vice chairman of NM Rothschild merchant bank.
- Sigurd Reinton, director of NATS Holdings (public-private partnership of national air traffic control) and ex director (senior partner) at McKinsey.
- Heather Lawrence, non-executive director of NMC Healthcare until 2016 (a FTSE 250 company) and current member of the Dr Foster Global Comparators Founders Board.
- Adrian Masters, ex McKinsey, IBM and Pricewaterhouse-Coopers.
- Stephen Hay, ex KPMG.

So Monitor is intended as an independent regulator in the NHS, which will police competition in the NHS and make decisions about hospital trusts which go bust. Does this really look to you like an independent set of people or is it likely, in view of their backgrounds, that they will make pro-marketisation and pro-privatisation decisions? This is what you might describe as **regulatory capture**.

Whilst Cameron pacified us that there would be no switch to an insurance-based model (although he wants to 'drive the NHS to be a fantastic business'), former health secretary **Jeremy Hunt** did not agree. It was hard to imagine what could be worse than Andrew Lansley. But his replacement was exactly that - the man **officially on record as saying that the NHS should be privatised.**

Back in 2005, Hunt co-authored, with others including Michael Gove, Tory MEP Daniel 'the NHS is a 60-year-old mistake' Hanaan and Greg Clark, a book called *Direct Democracy* in which they called for the NHS to be dismantled.[16] It's touching to think that a few years ago, in freezing winter, a then unknown MP by the name of Jeremy Hunt joined constituents for a candlelit vigil outside Parliament to highlight that his local hospital - the Royal Surrey in Guildford - was threatened with closure. Even the leader of his party, an apple-cheeked, smooth-faced, young David Cameron, brow as yet unfurrowed by the ordeals of being PM, dropped by to lend his support.[17] One might be forgiven for thinking that this is a classic case of the corrupting effect of power. In fact, this rank hypocrisy is quite prevalent with the same MPs, who voted in favour of the HSCA, protesting against hospital cuts and closures in their own constituencies. MPs are still spooked by the 'Kidderminster effect' after Dr Richard Taylor, running as an independent to reinstate the local A&E, won this seat in 2001 with a majority of 18,000 and was even re-elected in 2005.

The Act effectively paves the way for the piecemeal privatisation and break-up of the NHS. Now that the starting gun has been fired, the race to the bottom has officially begun. In October 2012, £262 million of NHS services (mainly community services) drew bids from 37 private companies. This was described as the **'biggest act of privatisation ever seen in the NHS'**.[18] In 2013, the Coalition planned to force a further £750 million of services to be opened up to competitive bids. A total of 105 private firms were approved for Any Qualified Provider (AQP) status. *The Guardian* highlighted some of the winners in this wave of privatisation:

InHealth was authorised to start operating in 95 places. InHealth earns about £80 million a year from the NHS but plans services at 100 extra locations.

Care UK planned to increase the £190 million a year it earns from NHS patients through 35 new contracts.

Specsavers won adult hearing contracts in at least 33 places.

Virgin Care was awarded AQP status in ten areas for which it applied. It planned to offer dermatology, ophthalmology, ultrasound, podiatry, back and neck pain services and fracture clinics.

BMI Healthcare has begun winning contracts to provide MRI and ultrasound scans.

Plasma Resources UK, which turns plasma into blood products, was privatised and sold to US private equity company Bain Capital; literally a case of Dracula in charge of the blood bank![19]

Unsurprisingly, the *Financial Times* reported that private sector companies are engaged in an arms race to win NHS contracts.[20] Subsequently, an estimated £2.6 billion worth of contracts were awarded to profit-driven companies, such as Bupa, Virgin Care and Care UK. **Circle** was the biggest winner with two contracts worth nearly £300 million. **Bupa** won a contract worth £235 million for musculoskeletal services.[21]

Analysis by the Institute of Fiscal Studies and the Nuffield Trust think-tank showed that the slice of the NHS budget going to non-NHS providers (private and voluntary sector) rose from £5.6 billion in 2006-07 to an estimated £8.7 billion in 2011-12 and has now topped £10 billion for the first time.[22]

The DoH's own figures reveal that private sector outsourcing reached nearly £9 billion in 2015-16, or 8 per cent of the budget, having doubled from 2009-10 when it was around £4 billion (or 4 per cent).

A **£1 billion contract** (later reduced to £800 million) for community health services in Cambridgeshire, which attracted bids from Virgin, Circle and Serco, was eventually awarded to an NHS consortium.[23] The contract trumped the value of similar arrangements made with Serco and Virgin to run services in

Suffolk (£140 million) and Surrey (£500 million). However, this is not the only contract of this magnitude. Whole service areas are now being offered up. In 2014, a **10-year contract for cancer services** and end of life care in Staffordshire across four CCGs - together worth £1.2 billion - was tendered but eventually collapsed.[24]

8 reasons why privatisation matters...

- NHS marketisation experiences demonstrate that markets do not work well in healthcare.
- This is further demonstrated by market-based healthcare systems internationally.
- Private providers cut costs (and therefore quality) - by cutting wages (not bound by national wage structures) and staff.
- Private providers are accountable only to shareholder profits cf. public ownership.
- Tendering will lead to fragmentation as opposed to genuine integration of care.
- The bidding process itself is hugely flawed and inefficient.
- Commercial confidentiality allows companies to hide behind a firewall of secrecy despite the public interest at stake.
- Ultimately, it will mean going down the road of private health insurance.

Section 75 is the key part of the Act. The Section 75 regulations pertain to the application of competition within the NHS. However, they caused a furore because they were latched on after the Act had been passed by Parliament. Keep Our NHS Public prepared a parliamentary briefing for MPs likely to be bamboozled by the chicanery of corporate law, having sought legal opinion from David Lock QC. This briefing surmised that the Section 75 regulations close down the current option of an **in-**

house commissioning process, even if local people wish it. This option was taken in a number of cases, including *since* the passage of the Act. Ministers confirmed that such arrangements were legal and would not give rise to challenge under **EU procurement law**: 'The regulations sweep all existing arrangements between NHS bodies, and just about all commissioning done by the CCGs, into a market framework - and thus into the remit of **EU competition law**. Once this is triggered, private providers gain rights which make halting their encroachment financially - and thus politically - virtually impossible.'[25]

Confused yet? Well let's think of an example. If your local CCG is deciding who will provide physiotherapy services, it may feel that the local hospital is doing a good job and should therefore continue. Instead, EU competition law will be applied to the tendering of all NHS contracts regardless of whether CCGs see fit or not, with the regulator Monitor having the power to enforce this. This means that **CCGs are forced to tender out contracts for fear of litigation.**[26] Virgin won a £2 million cash settlement from the NHS over a failed contract bid citing concerns over the tendering process. In fact, millions of pounds are already being wasted on legal fees in these tenders.[27] Labour uncovered that **the legal fees to comply with one clause of the Act cost CCGs £77 million a year.**[28]

This gives the lie to the government's claims that clinicians will be in control of decision-making. Of course, **the usual false assurances** were given...

Andrew Lansley: 'There is absolutely nothing in the Bill that promotes or permits the transfer of NHS activities to the private sector.' (13/3/12)

Andrew Lansley's letter to CCGs:

I know many of you have read that you will be forced to fragment services, or put them out to tender. This is absolutely not the case. It is a fundamental principle of the

Bill that you as commissioners, not the Secretary of State and not regulators - should decide when and how competition should be used to serve your patients' interests. (12/2/12)

Simon Burns MP: '...[I]t will be for commissioners to decide which services to tender...[T]o avoid any doubt - it is not the Government's intention that under clause 67 [now 75] that regulations would impose compulsory competitive tendering requirements on commissioners, or for Monitor to have powers to impose such requirements.' (12/7/11)

Lord Howe: 'Clinicians will be free to commission services in the way they consider best. We intend to make it clear that commissioners will have a full range of options and that they will be under no legal obligation to create new markets...' (6/3/12)

So how does this work in practice? Well the tendering of the NHS Direct telephone service is a good example. It has been 'broken up among 46 bidders for local 111 services, paid only 30% of the old cost per call', leading to contracts going bust whilst under-qualified operators (relying on simplistic algorithms) divert patients inappropriately to A&E.[29] Welcome to the wonderful world of markets!

Had enough yet? Well it only gets worse. Cost is the main consideration for CCGs in the tendering process both due to limited budgets and an obligation to seek value for taxpayer money. Larger companies tend to significantly under-cut on their bids. This strategy is known as a loss leader and is employed because they can afford to take a hit up front and recoup losses in future. However, as one CCG head confided to me, healthcare is not toilet paper. Lower cost simply means lower quality. As the journalist Polly Toynbee puts it, 'more for less' is Toryspeak for less and private. **Serco underbid the NHS trust's best price by £10 million on their £140 million contract for community health services in Suffolk. The result has been staff lay-offs and repeated concerns over poor performance.** Serco has temporarily pulled out of clinical services in the NHS and will focus on non-clinical services.

Furthermore, the bidding process is rigged in favour of these larger companies. The simple reason being that a multinational has the resources needed for the complex and costly bidding process whilst smaller organisations - often public or voluntary sector - do not. **The abandoned competition to run George Eliot Hospital cost £1.78 million** with £771,000 going to management consultancies.[30] The tender for the massive Cambridgeshire contract for community services will cost £800,000.[31] I have seen first-hand the time, money and effort poured into bidding for a local GP surgery. All of this would be better used for the benefit of patient care.

The knock-on effect is that smaller competitors, such as charities and co-ops, are edged out, with the result that a cartel develops. This phenomenon can be seen in outsourcing across various sectors. In other words, public sector monopolies - one of the supposed motives for privatisation - are merely replaced by private sector oligopolies.

As for the idea of empowering doctors, only a small number will be on the boards of CCGs. Some of these doctors are entrepreneurial types. Hence why **426 (36 per cent) of the 1179 GPs in executive positions have a financial interest in a for-profit private provider** beyond their own general practice - a provider from which their CCG could potentially commission services, according to the *BMJ*.[32]

Commissioning Support Units - set up to advise CCGs on how to spend most of the NHS budget - **could be spun-off and privatised**.[33] The usual suspects including Serco, UnitedHealth and McKinsey would likely bid to take them over. So these multinational companies (rather than clinicians) will advise CCGs on how to purchase services from the same private companies. It's a small world!

Even the American defence giant and international arms

company **Lockheed Martin** considered bidding and attended an NHS England meeting.[34] *The Guardian* has revealed the existence of a **Commissioning Support Industry Group (CSIG)** comprising UnitedHealth, McKinsey, KPMG, Capita, EY and PwC jockeying for commissioning contracts. CSIG receives regular briefings from senior NHS managers. UnitedHealth chairs the group and one of their lobbyists, Dr Chris Exeter (previously worked 'on non-health matters for Low Associates, a lobbying firm run by Sally Low, wife of…Andrew Lansley'), helps to coordinate meetings.[35]

NHS England has set up a lead provider framework for commissioning support services meaning that only approved suppliers can provide these services. This was drawn up by CSIG. Those that have made the cut include Optum (the UK division of American healthcare and insurance giant UnitedHealth), Capita and nationwide NHS Commissioning Support Units. The supply chain companies include the big four accountancy firms and commercial lobbying firms, such as Hanover. Hanover's clients include UnitedHealth, Hospital Corporation of America, the American Pharmaceutical Group (a US pharmaceutical lobby group) and Alliance Medical.[36]

Hence the corporate consortium eMBED, consisting of health information business Dr Foster, advisory firm Mouchel Consulting, accountancy firm BDO and consultancy Engine, won the contract to provide commissioning support services to 23 CCGs.[37]

Foundation Trusts are now allowed to earn 49 per cent of their income from treating private patients. This was previously capped at about 2 per cent. Hospitals are thus preparing to ramp up private patient work to increase incomes in the constraints of the current financial climate. Great Ormond Street Hospital anticipated an extra £11 million from treating private patients in 2013 compared with 2010 - that's a 34 per cent increase. Imperial College Healthcare was expecting an extra £9 million over the same period - a 42 per cent rise. According to a 2017 report in The Times, the Royal Marsden will earn 45% of its income from private patients and other non-NHS sources. Several other trusts, including University College, Royal Brompton, Moorfields, Papworth, Royal Surrey County and Chelsea and Westminster hospitals have all experienced soaring private patient incomes since the passage of the Act.

Across England, there has been **a 10 per cent increase in revenues from private patients compared with 2010.** Out of 146 Foundation Trusts, 40 plan to open private patient units.[38,39] Overt privatisation of hospitals - as with Circle taking over Hinchingbrooke Hospital - is politically toxic. So instead we get covert privatisation.

We have already been given a taste of this new NHS with the arrival on our shores of **Hospital Corporation of America (HCA) - one of the world's largest private healthcare companies**. HCA, co-owned by **Bain Capital**, whose profits helped fund **Mitt Romney's** presidential campaign, is looking to expand further into the NHS. HCA already caters for around half of all private patients in London. NHS England has come under fire after switching gamma knife contracts from the NHS to services run by HCA and Bupa.

Interestingly, private healthcare does not seem to operate along the lines of the idealised Adam Smith universe that neoliberals envisage. The Competition Commission's report - 'Private healthcare in central London: horizontal competitive constraints' - focused on the lack of competition and overcharging in the private healthcare market. The Centre for Health and the Public Interest published a report in 2013 warning that 'greater use of for-profit providers as a result of the Health Act is likely to substantially increase the amount of healthcare fraud in the NHS'. This would specifically be through overcharging to maximise shareholder returns. *The Independent* points out that **'HCA had to pay more than $1.7bn in fraud settlements in the**

US in 2003 after admitting 14 felonies'. [40]

According to a *New York Times* investigation, the factors behind HCA's rapid growth included more revenue from insurance companies, patients and Medicare through 'much more aggressive billing' and reducing expenses.

Step Seven: Plot against the NHS

It is therefore worth considering aiming over a period to end the state provision of healthcare for the bulk of the population, so that medical facilities would be privately owned and run, and those seeking healthcare would be required to pay for it.
Central Policy Review Staff document, 1982

Now if I told you that we have not even got to the most remarkable part of this story then you'd probably think I was lying. But you'd be wrong. Pretty much everything in this narrative was hatched in **a series of think-tank documents from the 1980s** - that something can be so faithfully executed over 30 years is a testament to Machiavellianism.

A frequent rejoinder has been that the concept of NHS privatisation is conspiracy theory - a label seemingly used to tar any argument with a batsqueak of paranoia. The argument goes that the popularity of the NHS would translate as electoral suicide if any government dared even contemplate dismantling the NHS.

However, privatisation plans for the NHS date back at least to Thatcher's first term. Central Policy Review Staff documents from 1982 proposed introducing education vouchers, ending state funding of higher education, freezing welfare benefits and an insurance-based health service. In fact, the original version went further and suggested compulsory charges for schooling alongside 'a drastic reduction in resources going to the public sector' and full-cost university tuition fees. With regards to the NHS, it stated that, 'It is therefore worth considering aiming over a period to end the state provision of healthcare for the bulk of the population, so that medical facilities would be privately owned and run, and those seeking healthcare would be required to pay for it'.[1]

Nigel Lawson, then energy secretary, said that this report caused 'the nearest thing to a cabinet riot in the history of the Thatcher administration'. The unpalatable nature of this proposition may help explain why think-tank documents from the late eighties such as Oliver Letwin and John Redwood's *Britain's Biggest Enterprise* and Madsen Pirie's *The Health of Nations* for the Adam Smith Institute recommended a piecemeal approach.

This is compatible with the approach endorsed by the Ridley Plan on nationalised industries in 1977:

> The process of returning nationalised industries to the private sector is more difficult than ever. Not only are the industries firmly institutionalised as part of our way of economic life, but there is a very large union and political lobby wanting to keep them so. A frontal attack upon this situation is not recommended. Instead the group suggest a policy of preparing the industries for partial return to the private sector, more or less by stealth. First we should destroy the statutory monopolies; second we should break them up into smaller units; and third, we should apply a whole series of different techniques to try and edge them back into the private sector.[2]

Dr Lucy Reynolds and Professor Martin McKee have charted this journey:

> [In the late 1980s]...a conference attended by Conservative politicians, NHS senior managers and think-tank advisors set out a seven-step plan to alter the NHS... In 1988, the pro-market Centre for Policy Studies published a series of short studies exploring this agenda...One study was published as a pamphlet entitled **'Britain's biggest enterprise'** by **Conservative MPs Oliver Letwin and John Redwood**.[3]

Here is an excerpt from 'Britain's biggest enterprise':

> Might it not, rather, be possible to work slowly from the present system towards a national insurance scheme? One could begin for example, with the establishment of the NHS as an independent trust, with increased joint ventures between the NHS and the private sector; move on next to the use of 'credits' to meet standard charges set by central NHS funding administration for independently managed hospitals or districts; and only at the last stage create a national health scheme separate from the tax system.[4]

It is worth noting that, around this time, Letwin and Redwood headed NM Rothschild bank's international privatisation unit and that Letwin had published a book called *Privatising the World* with a foreword by Redwood. (Just in case you're in any doubt as to the intentions of this dastardly duo and the Tories more generally towards the NHS, as some media commentators seem to be.)

Oliver Letwin has a Nostradamus-like tendency (or perhaps these are simply self-fulfilling prophecies when you are pulling the strings). *The Independent* reported in 2004 that Letwin told a private meeting the **NHS will not exist within 5 years of a Conservative government**. Two weeks previous, Letwin's plans for massive cuts to public spending were also leaked.[5] It is worth highlighting that this was long before any hint of a financial crisis. Both reports were, of course, strenuously denied!

In 1988, Madsen Pirie co-authored a paper called 'The Health of Nations' for the Adam Smith Institute.[6] This anticipated future reforms from the internal market, public-private partnerships, foundation trusts and outsourcing through to user charges and expanding private insurance.

The HSCA itself has been gestating for years and can be directly traced back to a speech Lansley made in 2005. The speech drew on his formative experiences as a civil servant involved in utility privatisations. **Lansley had been private secretary to Norman Tebbit when Tebbit was privatising BT**. As Nicholas Timmins documents in *Never Again: The Story of the Health & Social Care Act*, the full details emerged in 2007 in a white paper entitled 'NHS Autonomy and Accountability'. Right there, in the rubric, was the proposal for the private sector to bid for NHS work with no cap on the share they might secure. The other keynote ideas were already in place too - an NHS commissioning board with GPs in the driving seat, a new economic regulator to promote competition and all hospitals to become foundation trusts.[7]

In light of all this, the admission in 2015 by senior Tories on the front page of *The Times* that the NHS reforms were their biggest mistake has to be seen as a cynical election ploy![8] This article claimed that David Cameron did not understand the reforms. Either that or he is complicit in knowingly destroying our NHS. Guilty or incompetent? Whichever it is, he did not come out of this well. This may help to explain how he had the nerve in his conference speech in 2014 to state that he cares deeply about the NHS because it looked after his disabled son Ivan.

The genesis of current reforms can be traced back to the World Economic Forum (WEF) at Davos. In 2012, the WEF produced two reports looking into transforming global healthcare systems in the context of the aftermath of the financial crisis. The first report examined options including:

> various forms of rationing and shifting the cost burden onto individuals and employers through, for example, mandatory private insurance, or at the other end of the spectrum, increasing tax revenue. A third option, raising healthcare productivity through delivering more services with fewer resources would, it was argued, 'go a long way to ensuring their financial sustainability' whilst avoiding the 'fierce political contest' inherent in making either of the first two choices.

The report also explored the reduction in high cost channels such as hospitals in favour of low cost ones such as home-based, patient-driven self-care. The second report mapped out various potential scenarios.

As Stewart Player outlines:

Simon Stevens himself, who at that time was head of UnitedHealth's Global Division, acted as Project Steward of the Steering Board for the first WEF report, working with chief executives of leading healthcare companies including Apax Partners, Novartis, Merck, Medtronic and Kaiser Permanente, as well as the Directors of Health at the World Bank, the WHO, and the European Commission.

Not only are the prescriptions of these reports replicated in the Five Year Forward View (FYFV) - the current 5-year plan for the NHS - but some of the personnel of the WEF's healthcare groups have graduated to become Sustainability and Transformation Partnerships (STP) leaders. Player describes how the participants amount to a Who's Who of UK health policy leaders including Alan Milburn, Dame Julie Moore, Mark Newbold, Sir Robert Naylor, Sir Bruce Keogh, Niti Pall, Paul Bate, Paul Corrigan and Nick Seddon as well as representatives of UK private healthcare companies and two MPs - Stephen Dorrell and Liz Kendall.

As Player notes:

Kees Van der Pijl suggested that the WEF had reached the status of a true International of Capital, and that the 'organisation stood out as the most comprehensive planning body of the transnational capitalist class', where 'concepts of control are debated, and if need be, adjusted on a world scale', and whose aim is 'enhancing competition to the full and eliminating whatever niches remain protected from the full discipline of capital'.[9]

A 2017 WEF report reaffirmed plans of diverse stakeholders to overhaul global healthcare systems. These so called diverse stakeholders are almost all US global companies with the exception of Japanese corporation Takeda.

Step Eight: Brew the Perfect Storm

This is just the beginning. The NHS is being transformed into an umbrella for private provider purchasing, reduced to an insignia with enormous brand recognition. It's all very well for Theresa May to reassure us that the NHS remains free at the point of delivery (for the time being) funded by general taxation. But this is of little solace when the cost to the taxpayer has become exorbitant, whilst the private sector is enriched beyond measure.

In the wake of the 2008 financial crisis, the Brown government commissioned McKinsey & Company to propose strategies for reducing NHS expenditure. Never let a crisis go to waste so they say. McKinsey heeded this advice and produced a report 'Achieving World Class Productivity in the NHS 2009/10-2013/14: Detailing the Size of the Opportunity'. This recommended shedding up to 10 per cent of staff, i.e. 135,000 people, and led to the efficiency savings dubbed the Nicholson challenge. Nicholson's intolerant response to those opposing NHS reforms was: 'There are people in the service who essentially hate all this [i.e. Lansley's plans]. My view is that they should go.'

The looming NHS performance crisis is already unfolding, with projected NHS efficiency savings of £40 billion up to 2020. *The Telegraph* reports that as many as one in five hospitals are facing closures of some kind, A&Es and maternity wards are being shut down and thousands of NHS staff have been made redundant with waiting lists inevitably going up.[1] The *Daily Mail* even launched its own Save Our Hospitals campaign.

The dire situation in nursing exemplifies the chaos. Whilst the government cuts nurse training places, hospitals are forced to hire more expensive agency nurses, often from abroad. Likewise, numbers of district and community nurses are plunging, with district nurse numbers having halved since 2010.[2]

All of which highlights the hypocrisy at the heart of the NHS reforms. Theresa May and Jeremy Hunt talk about patient choice, improving standards and empowering healthcare professionals. Yet their policies enact the opposite through cuts, closures, sacking staff and privatisation. They may trumpet the slogan 'No decision about me without me' but what about the decision to privatise the NHS? I do not recall this decision being made with our consent.

The unravelling or how it will play out...

1) PFI debts will be a major factor in NHS trusts being allowed to 'go bust'.
2) Efficiency savings - or cuts - will be extended for years to come. This is a common fate of public sector organisations in which they are starved of cash and deliberately run into the ground. At which point, privatisation is conjured up as the unavoidable panacea.
3) Compulsory competitive tendering of contracts to Any Qualified Provider leads to cherry-picking. This means that high-volume, low-risk healthcare is picked off by private firms leading to unbundling of services and therefore a smaller pot of money to provide comprehensive healthcare, which in turn leads to increased rationing.

Think of your local hospital. This hospital is paid for the treatments and services it provides. It makes money from straightforward procedures like cataracts or hip and knee replacements. This money is then used to pay for expensive and risky healthcare like emergency medicine and intensive care. However, when the former has been cherry-picked by companies like Virgin and Serco then this money is permanently siphoned off out of the system leaving less to pay for the latter. To give one example, Circle had taken 30 per cent of the market share for hip, ankle and knee operations in the Bath area from 2010-11.[3] This, in turn, destabilises local health economies. So when David Cameron and Theresa May have stood at the dispatch box and stated that it does not matter who provides healthcare as long as it is free at the point of delivery then this is extremely misleading. And they both know it.

Furthermore, competitive tendering leads to fragmentation rather than integrated care - the buzzword of policy wonks.[4] Take the diabetic care pathway, which requires complex coordinated management - foot and eye care, diet and lifestyle education, optimising of blood sugar control and medication, monitoring of other risk factors like blood pressure and cholesterol. If this is fragmented amongst different providers (often not communicating with each other) then the quality of care deteriorates. Ideally this care should all be carried out by one provider. It makes much more sense to have collaboration rather than competition in healthcare.

Once you combine all of the above factors then you have a perfect storm in which the NHS withers away. Rationing of care is already accelerating. A *BMJ* survey showed that **one in seven CCGs have brought in new restrictions over what treatment people can get**, including those for recurrent migraines, new barriers to joint replacement and cataract operations.[5] In some areas, only one cataract is removed. Apparently one eye is enough! **A CCG in Devon even announced that obese patients and smokers would be denied all routine surgery, shoulder surgery would be restricted for all patients and hearing aids would be available for only one ear not two.**[6] This has been partially reversed. Some other CCGs have announced similar restrictions. Rationing and funding decisions can then be ascribed to doctors on CCGs rather than blamed on the government.

Rationing will become more widespread until we have a two-tier system in which the haves will be forced to take out private insurance and the have-nots will be looked after by a third-class health service. This is how you privatise the NHS by stealth.

PFI claimed its first scalp during the summer of 2012. **South London Healthcare Trust (SLHT) became the first NHS trust to go bust** after debts started accumulating at a rate of £1.3 million per week.[7] In fact, there are **two PFI hospitals in SLHT with a combined projected cost of £2 billion** - the Queen Elizabeth in Woolwich and the Princess Royal in Bromley, which will cost the NHS £1.2 billion alone, more than ten times what it is worth.[8] SLHT has the dubious honour of being the first trust to enter the Unsustainable Providers Regime. It was then announced that neighbouring Lewisham's A&E and maternity services would be sacrificed - presumably in order to keep servicing PFI repayments - despite Lewisham being a solvent, well-managed standalone trust. Based on precedents, the downgrading of emergency and acute care services is often the precursor to shutting down the whole hospital.

The Trust Special Administrator did not count on the Save Lewisham Hospital campaign. The turnout was estimated at 25,000 at its second demonstration. To think, there were only a handful of people at the first organising meeting. The campaign, aided by 38 Degrees, took Jeremy Hunt to the High Court and won. **A judicial review ruled that government plans were illegal.**[9] This sets an important legal precedent that when PFI trusts are bankrupt, they should not be restructured at the expense of their neighbours. Ever the bad losers, the Tories tried to change the law, handing special administrators enhanced powers for restructuring hospital trusts so that they will be unencumbered in future.[10]

The restructuring plans for SLHT demonstrated that **an NHS trust could be dismantled in as quickly as 18 weeks**. The sobering lesson is that, if a successful hospital like Lewisham is in danger of being downgraded, then no hospital is safe. NHS trusts should not be restructured through no fault of their own - leading to mergers, closures and shrinkage - when neighbouring trusts incur deficits. And as we have seen before, these deficits are often incurred through factors beyond their control like PFI payments indexed higher with each year. SLHT is a test case that can be rolled out across the country. There are now tens of NHS trusts in danger of going bust, with PFI debts as a major contributory factor.[11]

Coming soon to a hospital near you

NHS North West London has made the decision to downgrade four A&Es with plans to virtually close down over 300 beds at Charing Cross and near total closure of inpatient care at the 327-bed Ealing Hospital. This means there will be **no A&E for the boroughs of Hammersmith & Fulham, Ealing and Brent - a population of 750,000, or a city the size of Leeds**. The initial plans envisaged 'almost 1,000 bed cuts by 2015 in North West London, averaging 28 per cent cuts across all eight West London boroughs. This includes drastic cuts...of around a third of beds in three hospitals set to carry the additional workload when the A&Es are closed - Chelsea & Westminster, West Middlesex and Northwick Park'.[12]

Without investment in local community and GP services, this is surely the recipe for pushing already overstretched resources to breaking point. NHS North West London executives have been forced to admit publicly, 'there are **NO concrete plans to establish alternative, community-based services** to take the place of the axed hospitals'.[13]

Around 55 per cent of the Charing Cross site and 45 per cent of the St Mary's site will be sold off. The Naylor Review recommends the disposal of NHS land and assets worth billions to generate investment through public-private partnerships. The sale of NHS land and property is irreversible.[14] At the same time, Imperial College Healthcare Trust plans to double its private patient income.

Yet there is money to be made, even when it comes to these closures. Big four accountancy firms, big three management consultancies and magic circle law firms are all being paid millions to advise on the setting up of Sustainability and Transformation Partnerships (STPs)s and Accountable Care Organisations (ACOs) (these will be covered in Chapter 10). *The Independent* reported £17.6 million being spent nationwide on management consultants for the STP restructuring that will lead to hospital and service closures. The true figure for all private contracts tendered for STP administration is likely to be much higher.

The ironically titled *Shaping a Healthier Future* reconfiguration for North West London paid a McKinsey-led consortium over £7 million alone for the period between April and December 2014. Whilst PwC were paid over £1.5 million. The total spend on private contracts for this STP plan in the same 9-month time frame reached over £13 million.[15]

Camden CCG paid around £2.3 million in 2016 to McKinsey, Deloitte, Atos and other corporates for their services.

Similar plans for 'reconfiguration' or closure are unfolding in South West London - affecting Kingston, Epsom and St Helier hospitals - and are heading for East London. According to the *Daily Telegraph*, there are 66 implemented/planned A&E and maternity unit downgrades and closures across the country.[16]

Polly Toynbee summed it up nicely in *The Guardian*:

Follow the money: **£300m** is being tendered out by Monitor... to pay the administration costs of the 'failure regime' for **up to 60 bankrupt trusts over 4 years**...The notorious Mid-Staffordshire hospital has **£2.5m to pay McKinsey and Ernst & Young** as registered insolvency practitioners: these are just starter sums, with much more for reconfiguration. The failed South London trust has **£5m for McKinsey and Deloitte**, more to come. McKinsey is the big NHS player likely to get the lion's share, as Mid Yorks, North Yorks, Epsom, St Helier, Morecambe, Barking, Peterborough, the Friarage, Imperial,

Barts and scores more head towards the NHS Unsustainable Providers Regime.[17]

Breaking the allegiance and loyalty of staff is one of the important strategies for attacking a public sector organisation. This is often achieved through policies that demoralise and alienate them. Under the Coalition government, reforms to pensions mean that staff will effectively have to pay more, retire later and get less. There has been a year-on-year public sector pay freeze despite the independent NHS Pay Review Body recommending a 1 per cent pay rise for all NHS staff in 2014. Jeremy Hunt rejected this recommendation.[18]

Deloitte's 2014 report for the Royal College of General Practitioners highlighted chronic under-funding and under-investment underpinning the general practice crisis. The proportion of money going into general practice, as a percentage of the NHS budget, has been shrinking over many years. At the same time, demand is rising and more services are carried out by GPs. GPs have taken on more responsibilities, such as ordering tests and scans as well as more prescribing of medicines. Surgeries have extended opening hours and there has been a shift of hospital care into communities. For example, type 2 diabetes care used to be provided mainly by hospitals but now generally takes place in the community.

As a result, GP workloads are overstretched to breaking point and patients are frustrated as they are unable to book appointments. When I applied for general practice training in 2008, it was seen as an attractive career prospect and was oversubscribed. Fast forward to the present and junior doctors are put off by the prospect of burn-out. Many older GPs are retiring early due to stress. There is a serious recruitment and retention crisis. Unsurprisingly, there is a reliance on locum doctors. Instead of training sufficient numbers, the government's strategy will be to recruit more doctors from abroad and introduce physician associates.

Francis Maude - the former Conservative Party chairman and minister for the Cabinet Office - talks of running more hospitals and even emergency services outside the public sector. He floated the idea of mutual companies owned by employees. Maude also warned that more public sector jobs will be axed with further wage cuts.[19] Other possible models would include joint public-private ventures. As Professor Martin McKee points out, John Lewis is usually cited as the shining example of mutualisation although the reality is not always so benevolent. The Circle Health model may be more applicable with employees holding a minority stake whilst the real power lies with hedge funds. Unlike Germany, we do not currently have the legal safeguards to stop private equity buy-outs or corporate takeovers of mutualised hospitals. This is really a thinly-disguised shrinking of the public sector and privatisation by a different name.[20]

This is in keeping with David Cameron's 'Big Society' concept. However, as we have seen, the voluntary sector - charities, co-operatives, mutuals - does not appear to be the main beneficiary. The big society actually means a return to the pre-welfare state days, in other words to a Victorian world in which healthcare and welfare are not the responsibility of the state but of philanthropic organisations and individuals. This is clearly a regressive direction of travel for the country.

Step Nine: Redesign the Workforce

During the winter of 2015-16, junior doctors embarked on a series of rolling strikes over the threatened imposition of a new contract. The dispute would turn out to be the biggest industrial action of the twenty-first century in the UK and would drag on for a year. Nobody predicted that the junior doctors' strike would spearhead the anti-austerity movement. Or that the Conservatives would be in crisis less than a year on from their supposedly triumphant election victory. Dismayingly, it would all end with a whimper and not a bang.

The proposed contract planned to remove safeguards to prevent junior doctors from working hours in excess of the European Working Time Directive. It intended to redefine anti-social hours thus reducing pay banding for late evenings and weekends in order to supposedly fulfil an election pledge for a 7-day NHS. As a result, specialties with the greatest burden of anti-social hours, such as emergency medicine, would be adversely affected leading to a pay cut. The contract also discriminated against those who take time out; mainly women thus opening up gender pay gaps. It was even suggested that non-resident on-call doctors might be paid less than the minimum wage. This is what might be described, albeit hyperbolically, as the proletarianisation of a profession accustomed to the good life.

Lawyer Peter Stefanovic put it succinctly in a video blog. He went on the streets and asked passers-by: 'How would you feel if your boss came in one day and said - Saturday is the new Friday. 7 till 10 pm is the new afternoon. I'll pay you less and if you don't like it, I'm going to force you anyway.' Unsurprisingly, most people replied with unrepeatable epithets.

A new generation of young doctors were suddenly politicised culminating in marches in London and several cities in which thousands of doctors poured out on to the streets to vent their fury. Even so, newly formed campaign groups, such as NHS Survival, spoke of depoliticisation; patently an absurd position when taking on the government - nothing could be more political.

In spite of these protests, the government declined to re-negotiate the major sticking points whilst accusing the BMA of refusing to come to the table. Government privatisation cheerleaders were wheeled out. Allister Heath, now editor of *The Sunday Telegraph*, penned a column about how doctors are the 'victims of an NHS that's broken beyond repair'.[1]

Meanwhile, Mark Britnell, the former senior DoH civil servant, whom you may recall swished through the revolving door to work for KPMG and infamously advised a private equity conference that the 'NHS will be shown no mercy', wrote in *The Sunday Times* that the NHS is sick and requires a radical overhaul.[2]

Government claims around weekend safety were partially based on a paper, in which the authors warned that the reasons for increased mortality 30 days following admission from Friday to Monday inclusive are not clear. They added that it would be rash and misleading to infer that the deaths were avoidable.[3] Moreover, the government's case was severely damaged by various leaked documents including the government's risk register, which concluded that the 7-day NHS plan was not feasible with current funding, resources and staff.[4]

At one stage, Hunt's position looked untenable following potentially serious allegations around misinforming Parliament over weekend mortality statistics. Some in the media circus, scenting a potential kill in the offing with the scalping of Hunt, jumped on the bandwagon with a significant amount of coverage. However, the right-wing tabloids upped the ante; presenting junior doctors as greedy and caring only about their pay. *The Sun*'s editorials became especially notorious underlining the proximity of Jeremy Hunt to the Murdoch media empire.

Protracted industrial action enabled the government to smear doctors as endangering the welfare of the public. Junior doctors tried to point out that, in reality, the new contract endangered patient safety. Ultimately, the chosen model of industrial action was delivered with patient safety maintained. This was in keeping with international evidence showing that strikes, provided they are well organised, do not cause serious harm to patients. Inevitably, the strikes did cause short-term disruption. However, it is worth noting that thousands of procedures and operations are cancelled each week due to the perpetual NHS crisis manufactured by deliberate policy decisions.

In the summer of 2016, the BMA leadership proceeded to endorse a suboptimal amended contract and embarked on a nationwide roadshow to garner support prior to a referendum of the junior doctor body. Critics pointed out that this was arguably worse than the original and nearly 60 per cent voted against the new contract. This put the BMA in an untenable position, forced to call for more strikes over a contract that it had effectively supported.

After a year-long dispute, the BMA eventually blinked. It suspended industrial action and the contract was rolled out. The BMA stated that this was not capitulation but it was difficult to see it as anything else. Jeremy Hunt and the government certainly viewed it as a victory. Unsurprisingly, many junior doctors lost faith in the BMA leadership to deliver their will. One of the consequences was the emergence of a group called Doctors for Progress aiming to win as many seats as possible on the BMA Council.

The only hope left appeared to be a judicial review. Out of over 50,000 junior doctors, five going by the name of *Justice for Health* decided to take a leaf out of *Mr Smith Goes to Washington* and took the government to the High Court. Co-founder Dr Ben White described for me the collision between his training as a doctor and the world of politics pointing out that probity, honesty and integrity are paramount in medicine. It had been eye-opening, he said, to encounter 'a whole, new world' in which 'nobody tells the truth' and 'nothing is as it seems...evidence does not mean anything'.[5]

Ben was really speaking for the junior doctor body, which had been on a steep learning curve. As with the miners' strikes during the 1980s, they were up against the forces of global capital. Ben framed it as an evidence-based scientific approach versus an economic and political ideology. Ultimately this judicial review proved to be unsuccessful.

The government's line throughout had been consistent: 7-day NHS, even services, patient safety. On the other hand, doctors are accustomed to complex issues and the moral imperative to tell the truth however grey it might be. Normally this is a strength but here it would prove to be an Achilles' heel up against a reductively misleading black and white media narrative. They found themselves at the mercy of a largely corporate media, which ruthlessly edited their comments and was often aligned with government and establishment interests.

(In the same way, the entire austerity narrative has been seductively framed by the Conservatives and the right-wing media with simple stories and strong images. The national economy is portrayed as a household, which has overspent. The nation's credit card has been maxed out. Hence why the Conservatives need to clear up Labour's mess and fix the roof whilst the sun is shining. Of course, the reality that the crisis was due to a global banking crash not public overspending is immaterial - one would struggle to find a mainstream economist to endorse the government's view.)

The government's refusal to U-turn on the contract - as it has done on other issues - was telling. It intended to ram it through whatever the political cost. This was partly because the contract would set a precedent. New hospital consultant contracts are in the pipeline, which are likely to mean more work for less money.

The government has announced that it intends to reduce starting and final consultant salaries, increase out-of-hours work, remove the right to decline elective weekend work and abolish automatic pay progression.

The introduction of physician and nursing associates - who will carry out many of the roles and responsibilities of doctors and nurses - alongside the axing of the student nursing bursary represent other aspects of the redesign of a cheaper workforce. The reduction in the skill mix is part and parcel of the deprofessionalisation of medicine. This process originally started with Thatcher wresting day to day running of the NHS from doctors and matrons on hospital boards through the introduction of corporate style hospital management. The predictable response of junior doctors, threatening an exodus from the NHS in the event of contract imposition, was entirely in keeping with the ideological intent of the government.

The parameters of the junior doctors' contract debate were conveniently restricted by both sides to a dispute over pay and conditions. At the outset, this was understandable and could be explained away due to a lack of awareness of the bigger picture. Yet after immersal in a year-long struggle, it was extremely revealing that the medical establishment and junior doctor leaders were not prepared to highlight the bigger picture of privatisation. **In essence, the new junior doctor contract is about the redesign of the workforce to bring down the wage bill. This is intended to pave the way for privatisation because the wage bill is the most expensive overhead for any organisation.**

Only generalisation into a national movement to save the NHS from privatisation would have averted defeat. The BMA leadership would have done well to take heed of its own motto for the struggle - 'It's everyone's fight'. The correct strategy would have been to link up with all NHS staff and public sector workers. This would have included the student nursing campaign to reinstate the bursary - Bursary or Bust - and teachers, who were up in arms over plans to academise all schools. This could have become a launch pad for an anti-austerity mass movement.

In fact, the medical establishment was not prepared to ruffle too many feathers or rock the boat. And they were certainly not prepared to alienate the government. After all, the Royal Colleges have charitable status - something that could easily be revoked. At the tail-end of the dispute, Hunt's appointment of aide and senior DoH civil servant Charlie Massey as the new head of the General Medical Council just about summed up the cosiness of the medical establishment with the government - a relationship that few wished to endanger.

This was reflected in some media portrayals, which were overall relatively emollient for strike action. Admittedly, both Hunt and the tabloids were hysterical in their description of 'militant' doctors. Nothing could have been further from the truth. After all, many doctors are conservative in their opinions and significant numbers are Conservative voters.

Here, the history of the NHS is telling. It is worth recalling that the BMA was originally against the setting up of the NHS. Bevan infamously stated that he had been forced to stuff hospital consultants' mouths with gold - a reminder that doctors are part of the professional, well-to-do classes and the BMA is a professional body. Perhaps the most important lesson from the junior doctor struggle is that doctors alone will not save the NHS. Undoubtedly, though, they can play an important part in a coalition or broad-based movement if they choose to do so.

Political earthquakes

In parallel with the events described above, British politics was upended by seismic events. The dialectical reaction to the 2015 Conservative general election victory was the catapulting of rank outsider, backbencher and unapologetic socialist Jeremy Corbyn to the Labour leadership with a spectacular surge in party membership particularly amongst young people. Corbyn's victory signalled a decisive break from the neoliberal consensus of the main political parties for the first time in a generation. It reinvigorated the staleness of Westminster politics in which Cameron Conservatives, New Labour MPs and Orange Book Lib Dems were almost indistinguishable.

The ideological battle between the Parliamentary Labour Party (PLP) wing and the membership threatened to tear the party apart. The NHS amply illustrated these divisions. Corbyn and Shadow Chancellor John McDonnell were two of the earliest signatories to Allyson Pollock and Peter Roderick's NHS Reinstatement Bill. This Bill aimed to repeal the HSCA, reverse privatisation and marketisation, resolve the question of PFI debt and restore a publicly funded, provided and owned healthcare system. However, the majority of the PLP were not supportive and were still very much ideologically wed to the supremacy of deregulated free markets and the principles of public-private partnerships. For example, shadow health secretary (at the time) Heidi Alexander blocked the NHS Reinstatement Bill designating the Labour Party's official position as one of abstention.

The summer of 2016 would see the EU Referendum result in the decision to leave the EU. The fall-out of the Brexit vote culminated in a coup by Labour MPs intent on toppling Corbyn. Shadow health secretary Heidi Alexander was one of the main instigators. A few days after Alexander's resignation, a bizarre story surfaced in the health trade press authored by the editor of *Health Policy Insight*, Andy Cowper. The story partly attributed the source to Alexander's shadow health team.[6]

This story claimed that shadow chancellor John McDonnell had undermined Alexander's brief with a clandestine health policy review. The initial story stated that an NHS advisory group, including hard-left members, had been secretively set up. In reality, the group consisted of doctors, academics, a barrister and respectable campaigners. The group intended to advise Labour on the NHS, particularly around privatisation.

It supported the NHS Reinstatement Bill as the legislation to restore a public NHS. I happened to have a front-row seat to these events as I had been invited on to the McDonnell NHS think-tank.

In fact, Heidi Alexander had been present at two meetings in parliamentary rooms with a group of NHS campaigners. These meetings took place in January and April 2016. The Alexander team claimed that they had not been informed about the second meeting and only found out by chance. At the April meeting, the concept of an NHS think-tank was floated. The think-tank was subsequently set up but the newly constituted group never actually met with the Labour Party.

The story was then picked up by *The Guardian*'s health correspondent, Denis Campbell.[7] This inferred that the advisory group had been in breach of party rules due to the inclusion of individuals who were not Labour members. Yet Labour Party rules do not prevent it from consulting with experts. The article even named two of the members of the think-tank on this basis. That *The Guardian* felt it necessary to smear this advisory panel in an effort to undermine the leadership spoke volumes about both their indifference to a public NHS and their detestation of Corbyn and McDonnell.

As a result of the *Guardian* article, Emma Reynolds MP, then chair of the PLP's backbench health committee, got involved. She asked Labour's general secretary, Iain McNicol, to investigate whether McDonnell had broken party rules. The social media storm continued to unfold on Twitter. Dr Clive Peedell - previously co-chair of the National Health Action party - tweeted at Cowper to defend the advisory group. This led to Heidi Alexander intervening to broadly back up the version of events in the Cowper and Campbell articles. The original story was recirculated in a vitriolic opinion piece on Corbyn written by Alexander in *The Guardian* in August.[8]

It appears that this smear story was designed to partly justify the anti-Corbyn coup and to discredit serious efforts to restore a public NHS.

Alexander refused to attend junior doctors' picket lines and declined to wear a BMA badge when invited by a member of the BMA's Junior Doctors' Committee on the basis that patients would be disappointed. In marked contrast, Jeremy Corbyn and John McDonnell could be seen at the front of a junior doctors' demonstration at which they were invited speakers.

Yet, at the end of June, Alexander was billed to speak at the 2016 Health Plus Care conference - the largest national integrated healthcare conference sponsored by UnitedHealth's UK arm, Optum. Other invited speakers included Lord Andrew Lansley - the former Conservative health secretary and architect of the HSCA 2012 - and Blair's former advisor Paul Corrigan.

It appears that Alexander had inherited the New Labour health prospectus, which overlapped with Conservative policy. It supported health and social care devolution as well as integrated care. As previously described, New Labour had close links with private healthcare under Blair and Brown. Various New Labour health secretaries and ministers went through the revolving door to work for private healthcare interests.

Labour MP Owen Smith would ultimately challenge Corbyn in a second leadership contest. Alexander joined Owen Smith's leadership campaign as co-chair. On the Smith campaign, Alexander worked alongside her former advisor and ex lobbyist Ben Nunn. Nunn previously worked for health consultancy Incisive Health co-founded by Bill Morgan - former special advisor to Lord Andrew Lansley. Nunn also worked for MHP Communications, which is one of the UK's biggest PR and lobbying firms. Its healthcare clients have included blue-chip names like AstraZeneca, Bayer and Roche. Owen Smith's campaign manager was lobbyist John Lehal. Lehal was the founder and managing director of Insight Consulting Group with clients including pharmaceutical giants, such as Novartis.

Smith attempted to position himself as an NHS champion by highlighting privatisation. Yet Smith had spent 5 years working in big pharma, some of that as a corporate lobbyist. He was Head of Policy and Government Relations for Pfizer, renowned as the manufacturer of Viagra. Whilst at Pfizer, he lost a 2006 by-election. According to the *Telegraph*, Smith 'boasted that Pfizer had been "extremely supportive" of his aspirations to public office'.[9]

Smith went on to work as chief lobbyist in the UK for American biotech company Amgen. Whilst he was there, Amgen were battling a US investigation. They were eventually fined $762 million for 'pursuing profits at the risk of patient safety'.[10]

This begins to inform us of Owen Smith's world view. He came from a background of lobbying government on behalf of massive corporations. Soon after becoming a Labour MP in 2010, he stated that government ministers should offer more incentives for pharmaceuticals and warned that the use of cheaper, non-patent drugs by the NHS could affect the industry.[11]

It was therefore a remarkable transformation for Smith to position himself as a champion of ordinary people. So let's have a look at what he has said on the NHS in the past. He supported a Pfizer funded report in favour of patient choice. The report spelt out what was meant by choice - direct payments for services and easier access to private sector healthcare.[12]

On PFI, Owen Smith stated that, 'If PFI works, then let's do it...I'm not someone, frankly, who gets terribly wound up about some of the ideological nuances that get read into some of these things, and I think sometimes they are totally overblown.' On the use of the private sector in the NHS, Smith stated:

Where they can bring good ideas, where they can bring valuable services that the NHS is not able to deliver, and where they can work alongside but subservient to the NHS and without diminishing in any respect the public service ethos of the NHS, then I think that's fine. I think if their involvement means in any way, shape or form the break-up of the NHS, then I'm not a fan of it, but I don't think it does.[13]

To have, or not to have an NHS Commission: that is the question

BMA Junior Doctor Committee chair Johann Malawana - critiqued by a hostile media as an entrepreneur medic - curiously went on to set up The Healthcare Leadership Academy with some eyebrow raising appointments to its faculty. These included former Conservative health minister Dan Poulter, former Labour shadow health secretary Heidi Alexander, who was one of the main instigators of the coup against Corbyn, and Lord Patel, who headed up a House of Lords NHS Sustainability Committee that many campaigners feared might recommend charging and top-up payments.

This House of Lords NHS Sustainability Committee had been quietly launched. The committee members included Lord Norman Warner. Warner is one of a succession of health ministers who swished through the revolving door in order to advise private healthcare interests. Within minutes of the first evidence session of the Committee, here is what Lord Willis of Knaresborough asked Andrew Baigent, Director of Finance at the DoH:

I find it somewhat incredible, given that, with every modern healthcare system, we are facing issues of long-term sustainability, and given that you have to integrate health and social care into a single package, that you are doing absolutely no thinking about whether there are any items in both health and social care that we could remove from being free at the point of delivery and put on to a pay list. Is none of that thinking going on? If not, could we have your personal view as to whether we should be doing it?[14]

Ultimately this committee concluded that taxation is the most efficient way to fund the NHS. Nevertheless, the concept of a cross-party health and social care commission is still being lobbied for. In 2015, a campaign group called NHS Survival had been set up. It consisted of doctors, patients and campaigners. According to its website, it planned to lobby for the setting up of a commission on the future of the NHS. The executive members felt that the NHS had become a political football kicked around for short-termist gains. Their aim was to depoliticise it.

NHS Survival gained a remarkable level of traction very quickly. Some of its executive members went on to become very prominent in the junior doctor dispute. They arranged meetings with MPs. Gradually, the idea of the commission began to attract powerful sponsors. These included Alan Milburn, Norman Lamb and Stephen Dorrell.

However, such allies appeared to be strange bedfellows. As previously described, Milburn had been Blair's health secretary. He was one of the key architects of NHS privatisation in the New Labour years. He implemented the NHS Plan 2000 bringing in private providers as permanent fixtures in the NHS. Milburn also enabled the expansion of PFI into the NHS.

Stephen Dorrell was Conservative health secretary under John Major. Meanwhile, Norman Lamb was Liberal Democrat health minister under the Coalition government when the HSCA 2012 was introduced. Lamb, Milburn and Dorrell coordinated their calls for the commission.

On the Lords side, there were also powerful allies. These included Lord Prior, who was previously head of the attack dog Care Quality Commission. In December, Lord Norman Fowler, at one time Thatcher's health secretary, wrote an article in the *Daily Telegraph* supporting the commission and calling for a health insurance system. A similar piece appeared almost simultaneously on the ConservativeHome website.

Lord Fowler wrote that, 'Most radical of all, a Royal

Commission could try to settle the argument once and for all on whether it would be possible to move to an insurance system, with exemption for those unable to pay. This would have the huge advantage of taking much of the health bill out of public spending by the taxpayer.'[15]

Other supporters of a cross-party commission have included Labour MP Liz Kendall and Conservative chair of the Health Select Committee Sarah Wollaston. It should be noted that legislation is not necessary for the setting up of a commission if there is sufficient cross-party consensus. There have, of course, been NHS commissions in the past. However, the NHS privatisation programme appears to be entering the endgame. **In the current climate, it is not unrealistic to imagine that a cross-party commission could arrive at a set of recommendations including charging and insurance as solutions to the bogus debate around NHS affordability and sustainability.**

One possible scenario would see the government adopt these recommendations. The 'independent' and cross-party status of the commission would effectively grant the government a get out of jail card to avoid electoral suicide. Such recommendations would then be implemented so insidiously that they would hardly be noticeable to begin with.

Step Ten: Restructure the NHS into a US-style Insurance System

The opening up of NHS contracts, as a result of the HSCA 2012, has arguably not been as lucrative as envisioned for corporate and financial interests. The current phase of restructuring the NHS appears designed to create economies of scale (and therefore enhanced profit margins) ready for corporate takeover.

The government is currently introducing US style healthcare models known as Accountable Care Organisations (ACOs). Due to the furore around this, ACOs have been rebranded as Integrated Care Organisations. In order to achieve this, the NHS is being divided into 44 Sustainability and Transformation Partnerships (STPs). The concept that the NHS is no longer sustainable or affordable is largely a PR narrative spun by the private healthcare lobby despite the fact that international evidence demonstrates that public healthcare systems are the most cost-efficient. In this context, sustainability means £22 billion in efficiency savings (taking the total amount of cuts for the NHS to approaching £40 billion for this decade), whilst transformation means new models of care, some of which are linked to privatisation. Each STP entails the consolidation of several CCGs. Some STPs will then be rolled out as Accountable/ Integrated Care Systems (ACS/ICS) before presumably transitioning into ACOs.

ACOs originated in the US as a response to Health Maintenance Organisations (HMOs) - dominated by large insurance corporations and considered by many to be the most objectionable part of the US healthcare system:

The history of HMOs isn't exactly edifying, and includes routine denial of patients' access to medically necessary treatment, fighting claims, screening out the sick, paying exorbitant CEO salaries, and undertaking systemic fraud. And all while offering what is effectively low rent medical care with considerable hidden costs in the forms of top-ups and deductibles.[1]

Accountable care can also be viewed as an evolution or mutation of HMOs with supposedly friendly providers taking the lead instead of insurers. However, it now appears that: 'the insurance industry - companies like Aetna, UnitedHealth, Humana and Blue Cross - are taking a leading role in developing the model'.[2]

So insurance companies ran HMOs and are now in the driving seat behind the setting up of ACOs. UnitedHealth already has contracts with more than 800 ACOs across the US and has launched a national accountable care organisation available to employers.

So how does this translate into the NHS? Eight Accountable/ Integrated Care Systems (ACS/ICS) are being rolled out. Accountable Care Systems will mean that various parties - NHS trusts, councils, private companies - will be responsible for the administration and control of health and social care budgets as well as ultimately for the delivery of services. This dovetails with the devolution of regional health and social care budgets to local bodies as can be seen with the Devolution Manchester experiment. The sharing of budgetary savings is intended to align incentives in order to maximise efficiency.

However, the shift towards ACOs would likely see a single organisation responsible for all of the above. (The draft ACO contract published by NHS England in August 2017 envisages that a group of CCGs will contract with a single provider - the ACO - to provide defined services to people on a list maintained by NHS England - a note states 'persons resident on it [i.e. the Contract Area] will be entitled to register with the Provider or seek acceptance by the Provider as a temporary resident'.)

Notably, the ACO can be an NHS provider or a private

company, including a complex financial instrument known as a Special Purpose Vehicle (SPV). A separate 'Alliance Agreement' will allow the CCGs and provider to decide how the contract will be administered. DoH documents define new models of care as types of accountable care.[3]

These new models include the multispecialty community provider (MCP) and the integrated primary and acute care system (PACS). (The MCP is a predominantly out of hospital-based care model integrating primary care with community and mental health services. The integrated PACS is similar to the MCP but incorporates many hospital-based services. The same document states that both models are types of whole population provider and are forms of ACO. NHS England's 'New Care Model' programme includes 23 vanguards piloting MCP and PACS models.)

The government cites the Alzira model in Valencia, Spain as a template in which the Valencia government combined with the Ribera Salud corporate consortium financed, ran and delivered regional health services. In this context, ACOs can be seen as a form of public-private partnership going beyond PFI. Accountable care is also called managed or integrated care. As previously discussed, integrated care basically means restriction of access to expensive hospital or specialist care and the delivery instead of this care in the community. Intriguingly, it harks back to the fad for polyclinics under New Labour.

The government has justified ACOs on the basis that they will abolish the internal market and competition. This would reduce fragmentation and enable improved, integrated care. As with previous justifications for reforms, this is proving to be a persuasive argument. However, both devolution and accountable care raise multiple concerns. For starters, how does one integrate privatised and means-tested social care with public, universal health care?

Two judicial reviews attempted to put the brakes on the

shift towards accountable care. Professor Allyson Pollock and colleagues, previously supported by the late Professor Stephen Hawking, pursued a judicial review on the basis that the absence of legislation (and parliamentary scrutiny) means that non-statutory, non-NHS bodies could run ACOs. In effect, there would be nothing to stop private healthcare or insurance companies from taking over - evidently a disturbing development completely divorced from the founding principles of the NHS. The second judicial review focused on the fact that one model of accountable care employs capitated or global fixed payments meaning that a total cap is imposed on the health and social care for all patients in a geographic area regardless of need or demand.

The repeal of the HSCA and the adoption of the NHS Reinstatement Bill would be the straightforward way of initiating the process of reversing privatisation and competition. **In fact, accountable care represents the consolidation of privatisation carried out by stealth without legislation.** ACOs would carve up the NHS into piecemeal segments ready for corporate takeover. As if to underline this danger, Nottingham and Nottinghamshire STP has awarded a £2.7 million contract to Capita and the UK arm of major US healthcare insurer Centene Corporation in order to develop the plans into an accountable care system.[4]

In essence, accountable care dovetails neatly with the massive programme of cuts and closures. Since 2010, over 60 NHS hospitals have experienced or are facing closures, mergers or downgrades according to the *Daily Telegraph*. Furthermore, NHS England previously announced that it intended to reduce the number of major A&E departments in England to between 40 and 70. This plan now appears to be on the back burner but it may resurface in the near future. *The Guardian* reports that 1 in 6 A&E departments are at risk of closure or downgrade. The *Health Service Journal* reports that 24 of 33 hospitals under discussion are likely to lose full A&E services. Chris Moulton, vice president of the Royal College of Emergency Medicine, described these plans as 'crazy'.[5] Such proposals for hospitals are in keeping with the Dalton Review's plans to create chains of super hospitals (more of this later).

Current bed to population ratios have plummeted below some Eastern European countries despite the UK being the fifth/ sixth biggest economy in the world. The winter of 2016/17 saw the British Red Cross declare a humanitarian crisis inside the NHS. The severity of recent winter crises indicate that such plans would be nothing less than disastrous and reckless. Shocking figures for the 2016 spring crisis revealed that some 66.5 per cent of the most serious ambulance Red-1 calls - where patients are not breathing or do not have a pulse - were responded to within 8 minutes against a target of 75 per cent.[6]

In 2015, 30,000 excess deaths were uncovered representing the largest increase in deaths in the post-war period. This analysis, published in the *Journal of the Royal Society of Medicine*, ruled out data errors, cold weather and flu as main causes and found that there was clear evidence of health system failures with almost all targets missed including ambulance call-out times and A&E waiting times. The authors also noted that the situation has been exacerbated by dramatic reductions in the welfare budget of £16.7 billion and in social care spending.[7] 10,000 additional deaths have also been reported in the first 7 weeks of 2018 compared to the same period in the previous 5 years.[8] **Overall, 120,000 excess deaths have been linked to austerity since 2010.**[9]

The very notion of care in the community is extremely problematic in the context of huge cuts to welfare and social care budgets. Over this decade, general practice has been chronically under-funded as a proportion of the NHS budget. Over 650 GP surgeries have closed, merged or been taken over since 2010. The Royal College of General Practitioners (RCGP) predicts up to a further 600 surgeries could close in the coming years.[10] Around 40 per cent of walk-in centres have closed since 2010.[11] At the same time, there are plans to reduce the number of GP surgeries from 7500 down to 1500 super hubs.[12]

This is already happening in my neighbourhood of Southwark in London, with the merger of 4 GP surgeries into the Nexus Health Group - an ominously corporate sounding name. The GP Forward View document proposes the creation of networks of federated GP organisations. Notably, David Cameron chose to make his first post-2015 election speech at just such a federation - the Vitality Partnership in Birmingham. Since renamed Modality, the federation told the Kings Fund that its 'super-partnership' model was actually a 'GP managed care organisation'.[13]

Privatisation

Meanwhile, privatisation expands in all manner of ways. Dorset GPs are offering a bespoke private service charging £40 for a 10-minute phone consultation, £80 for a 20-minute face to face appointment and £145 for 40 minutes with a GP.[14] At the England Local Medical Committees conference, a proposal was made for struggling GP practices to go private although it was voted down. Meanwhile, foundation trust hospitals are currently setting up private companies. These range from companies to provide private patient services to transferral of NHS staff to subsidiary companies.

Digital healthcare represents a new opportunity for corporates. Google DeepMind set up a partnership with the Royal Free NHS Trust resulting in the transfer of 1.6 million identifiable patient records to Google DeepMind in order to test its Streams application for the management of acute kidney injuries. The Information Commissioner has ruled that this data transfer was inappropriate.[15] Incidentally, back in 2014, the *Telegraph* revealed that the medical records of all NHS hospital patients between 1997 and 2010 had already been sold to insurance companies.[16] Google is far from alone. Big tech corporations, such as Apple, Facebook and Amazon, are also investing heavily in health startups, digital apps, healthcare data and medical research.

The NHS-funded GP at Hand, powered by private company Babylon, has now entered the market. It enables smartphone virtual consultations and if necessary face to face appointments at various clinic locations. However, patients are first required to deregister from their own GP. Furthermore, GP at Hand has recommended that certain groups may be 'less appropriate' including pregnant women, patients with complex needs, complex mental health problems, dementia, safeguarding needs, learning disabilities, drug dependence, end of life care and older, frail patients. This has triggered a storm of controversy over cherry-picking patients and undermining equitable access with consequent destabilisation of the income of other GP practices. There is also a separate Babylon private app - similar to Push Doctor - advertising fast-track access to GPs with a pay as you go service or a subscription fee.

The critical factor driving privatisation is the saturation of the US healthcare market forcing US corporations to expand globally. For example, Vernon Baxter from *Health Investor* magazine states that, 'The US market has been heavily invested into and there is a scarcity of assets...[the major US companies] have bought everything in North America and now American capital is looking at buying a lot of the assets in the UK and western Europe.'[17]

The NHS Improvement Business Plan 2016/17 proposed as priorities joint ventures and/or outsourcing of clinical services, joint ventures and novel financing for facilities and/or technology and private sector management models to support capability and leadership challenges.[18] Hospital Corporation of America (HCA) has formed HCA NHS Ventures, which are partnerships with NHS trusts to provide clinics and hospitals including state of the art cancer facilities at Guy's hospital and Harley Street at University College Hospital. Patients attending appointments at Guy's hospital are confronted by a HCA kiosk at the entrance of the brand new cancer centre. On leaving, they are likely to come across a HCA clinic operating underneath the Shard building. In fact, HCA has been given four floors of the brand new cancer centre with the rent effectively covering the mortgage of the entire building.[19]

HCA also operates strictly private hospitals in London, such as the Princess Grace and the Portland hospital. It is one of the biggest healthcare facility companies in the US with the UK arm as part of the Private Hospitals Alliance - a lobbying group supporting the role of private participation in the NHS. Some US companies have entered the UK market through acquisitions such as US hospital and clinic operator Tenet Healthcare acquiring Aspen Healthcare, which is an operator of private services in the UK. Tenet noted to investors that, 'privatisation of UK marketplace, given market inefficiencies and pressures on the NHS, should create organic and de novo opportunities'. Meanwhile, the exclusive Cleveland Clinic is reportedly exploring opportunities in the UK including NHS contracts.[20] Whilst IBM has taken over electronic staff records services from another US company - drug distributor and healthcare services company McKesson.[21]

In the West Midlands, the Dudley Clinical Commission Group has tendered a £5 billion contract over 15 years for a MCP. Dudley CCG's document entitled 'New Care Model Value Proposition' states that 'a review of experience from the creation of Accountable Care Organisations **in the United States** has fundamentally influenced our approach to evaluation'. They go on to say, 'we articulated the value of our programme using a similar framework to that used by **Bain & Co** to guide this submission'.

As the Public Matters blog put it: 'So a clear statement that the US model was the influence and the framework was from one of the "Big 3" US global management consultancies. **Bain & Co describe themselves as the leading consulting partner** to the private equity industry and its key stakeholders and as a strategic partner and active member of the World Economic Forum.'[22]

Personal health budgets: a Trojan horse

Personal health budgets are exactly what they sound like - a patient can use money directly for purchasing health and other services. For example, they might purchase a block of physiotherapy sessions for £500. Or they might feel that they would better use that money on gym membership. Or buying a bike. Personal health budgets have been used for personal care for many years. Pilots are on the verge of being rolled out to hundreds of thousands of patients and could be extended nationwide including for maternity and end of life care.[23] It's all about empowerment, right?

Wrong. They represent the **logical end-point of the journey with the self-paying consumer in a market for healthcare**. The real question is what happens when your personal health budget runs out. Easy, you top it up. Or not so easy if you don't have the money. In other words, they enable insurance for top-ups (co-payments). Hence why insurance companies like WPA and AXA PPP are reportedly enthusiastic. At the same time, Bupa has been busy preparing its own clinical guidelines and creating networks of doctors gearing up for this brave, new world. Personal health budgets undermine the fundamental NHS principle of equity of care. They are a Trojan horse for privatisation.

The publication of the Dalton review in December 2014, commissioned by the government, has looked at whether public or private companies could own and operate chains of hospitals. Case studies for this review included Spain and Germany, where privately-run public hospitals have expanded. Alternatively, this might pave the way for 'new conglomerations of super NHS trusts, some privately managed', which could entice private investors and even buy-outs from private equity groups.[24]

So we will have budget-holding patients under an NHS modelled on state insurance providers such as Medicare in the US, with CCGs acting as insurance pools - able to exclude undesirable patients, buying healthcare from private companies and making funding decisions supported by privatised commissioning support units. Top-up co-payments as well as care pathways and packages would then allow integration of this system with private healthcare insurance giants.

Although ministers, including Prime Minister Theresa May, continue to omit the P word, what is happening on the ground is clearly privatisation according to the **World Health Organisation definition of healthcare privatisation: 'a process in which non-governmental actors become increasingly involved in the financing and/or provision of healthcare services'.**

You see, the privatisation of the NHS affects us all. One bandies around the platitude that you never know when you will need the NHS. But as a fit young person, you don't seriously believe it. Until something happens, as I discovered in 2013 when I ruptured my Achilles tendon playing football - the textbook injury of the dilettante weekend sports-player. I was on crutches for 4 months under the care of the orthopaedic team and then required weekly physiotherapy for several months after. At the same time, my father - a retired consultant psychiatrist - was very unwell in hospital, requiring intensive care at one point. We have since both made a good recovery thanks to the NHS. To think that the government allied with the private healthcare sector wants to take the right to healthcare away from each and every one of us - when we are at our most vulnerable - makes my blood boil.

At the time, I was invited to a patient workshop at a large, central London teaching hospital at which one of the consultants spoke of the increasing numbers of patients and how this would be good news if only they were a business. The irony did not pass by unnoticed, as I thought to myself gosh you are a business in all but name. As a foundation trust, they are paid by throughput in a market-based system. They are free to make partnerships with companies and up to half their income can come from private patients.

As for general practice, the threatened abolition of the Minimum Practice Income Guarantee means that more than 100 surgeries, in deprived parts of the country, may have to close. This will be coupled with cuts to GP funding thus not taking into account the extra spending needed for deprived areas. I work in Tower Hamlets, where the life expectancy of our patients is 10-15 years shorter than other parts of London. Some practices could lose hundreds of thousands of pounds a year. Again, the result will be either closure or a massive reduction in what they can offer. It is likely that GP surgeries will be forced to merge, attracting private investment and facilitating takeovers.

New GP contracts are being converted to APMS (where contracts can be made with companies employing salaried GPs) to comply with competition rules. This means that **all GP contracts would then be tendered and are open to privatisation** and franchising.[25] APMS contracts last 5 years, which will also encourage short-term profiteering rather than long-term investment in public health. It will also spell the end of the traditional model of family doctors.

As if we do not already have enough to worry about, there is the prospect of Brexit.

Theresa May's hand-holding with Donald Trump is emblematic. May has refused to rule out the NHS as part of a free trade deal with the US. Meanwhile, Jeremy Hunt tweets that he wants the US and UK health sectors to work together. The post-Brexit Global Britain strategy will mean bilateral free trade agreements with bigger markets such as Trump's America, the European Union and China forcing the NHS and public services open to transnational corporations. It will also mean a bonfire of regulations around workers' rights, health and safety as well as environmental protections.

However, it should be noted that the NHS privatisation juggernaut is proceeding regardless of being inside or outside of the European Union. In fact, the Maastricht Treaty embodied the transition from a social democratic to a neoliberal model. The Maastricht Treaty applied monetarist control of inflation. Maastricht also imposed limits on government public spending. This was dictated through limits on government debt and deficit as a proportion of GDP. It is no coincidence that John Major's government ratified Maastricht and introduced PFI. The two are intimately connected. Once public spending was curtailed, governments turned to the financial sector for private investment of infrastructure. One of the consequences is that instead of public revenues being reinvested, private profits are siphoned offshore.

Remaining in the European Union would have also entailed being part of the **Transatlantic Trade and Investment Partnership (TTIP).** It is likely that post-Brexit trade deals will not be too dissimilar to the original TTIP model. Linda Kaucher has untangled the subtext of TTIP in an article for OpenDemocracy.[26] She explains that this EU-US trade agreement, like all 'trade agreements', is effectively an 'irreversible commitment made at the level of international law, i.e. beyond changes at the level of the UK government or the EU'. Financial services is a major force for the **liberalisation** of public services, opening them up to transnational investors and thus privatisation. When public services are committed to 'international trade agreements, the liberalisation of those services is then locked in', i.e. irreversible.

TTIP could give transnational corporations rights to:

- Operate without limits on activities, or on the number of transnational corporations that enter the sector.
- Same or better treatment than national companies.
- Rights to sue government in an international jurisdiction if

there is any attempt to limit rights or introduce regulation which might limit corporations' expected future profits. These are called **investor-state dispute settlements (ISDS)**.

ISDS allows corporate lawyers to sue governments in secretive, private courts. Other trade agreements have already facilitated countless examples of corporations suing governments over measures taken for the public good. Phillip Morris has sued the Australian government over plain packaging for cigarettes. A Swedish firm is suing the German government over the decision to ban nuclear power. Argentina was sued by international utility firms over freezing energy and water bills and has been forced to shell out over a billion dollars for this and other such claims.[27] In the first 16 years of the North American Free Trade Agreement, Canada, Mexico and the US 'faced 66 such claims costing several hundred million dollars in compensation and legal fees'.

ISDS essentially acts as a deterrent to prevent governments acting against corporate interests. The Labour Party has promised to repeal the HSCA but even so, deregulatory free trade deals would still lock in privatisation and might well mean that it would be too costly to renationalise NHS services. Labour have also vowed to exempt the NHS but this is not a straightforward matter due to complex legal mechanisms.[28]

CETA - the Comprehensive Economic and Trade Agreement - is the EU-Canadian trade deal. It includes a proposal for an Investment Court System or arbitration courts for investors. As Green MEP Molly Scott-Cato has written, all services will be subject to a liberalised trade system unless exempt although this slim exemption would appear to only apply to core government functions, such as law enforcement, the judiciary and central banking.

In fact, it is possible that the HSCA was originally drawn up with TTIP in mind. Health would then be the first sector to be *harmonised*, meaning that regulations will be aligned between the EU and US. However, regulatory 'harmonisation' with the US will be much broader. Another obvious target for 'harmonisation' is the European public broadcasting model. So the BBC, whose public duty is to inform you of what is in this book, could be next in the line of fire.

The HSCA is a centrepiece policy that has to be seen in the context of the wider Conservative project. The Tories have taken a wrecking ball to the public sector setting in motion the dismantling of the welfare state on a scale that Thatcher could scarcely have dreamt of. The chutzpah is breath-taking and one is left asking how they manage to get away with it. As the spectre of austerity sweeps through Europe, the social contract is being ripped up. The electro-shock therapy applied to Greece is an experiment that can be implemented elsewhere. After decades of wreaking havoc across the world, **neoliberalism writ large - in the form of privatisation, deregulation and shrinking the puiblic sector** - has come home to roost.

The NHS was created in the wake of World War II during a time of real austerity and shared suffering in a society based on communal values. As Peter Wilby has pointed out, this 'collectivism came naturally to people who had emerged from a devastating war that required patience, stoicism and personal sacrifice for the common good'. On the first day of the NHS, some doctors barricaded themselves in their offices anticipating a stampede. Instead patients formed an orderly queue.[29]

After 30 years of neoliberalism, we have a fragmented, atomised society of hyper-individualism. In other words, the collective ethos of the public sector comes into collision with the consumerist culture of instant gratification in which the concept of waiting is intolerable. As Wilby sums it up, 'Public services, free at the point of use, cannot work as goods and services offered through the private sector market do. They provide to all at low public cost what would otherwise be available only to some at high private cost…Nobody expects a bus to turn up at a time of their choosing as a taxi would.'

Are the NHS and the welfare state compatible with this new world? That's the question millions of people - particularly young people - are going to have to figure out for themselves. Bevan's vision was to ensure that healthcare was never again a commodity. Sadly we are regressing back to that pre-NHS world, where healthcare is distributed according to ability to pay rather than need. **The British public has not been consulted on this momentous decision that arguably affects each of us more than anything in our lives. These government policies, which will harm the health of an entire nation, carried out without the consent of the people, are nothing less than an act of betrayal.**

As Martin Luther King once said, **'Of all the forms of inequality, injustice in health care is the most shocking and inhumane.'**

Resistance is NOT futile. This is a call to arms.

One only has to look at the devolved countries to see the NHS in its original remit - as a publicly funded, publicly provided and publicly accountable service. Scotland has abolished the internal market after devolution.

The survival of the NHS is imperilled and it is on the verge of extinction. It's up to all of us.

What can you do?

- Retain our NHS as a publicly provided, publicly funded and publicly accountable service by supporting the **Campaign for the NHS Reinstatement Bill**: http://www.nhsbillnow.org
- Get involved with local NHS campaigns
- Arrange a local screening of **Michael Moore's** *Sicko*, *Sell Off* or the upcoming *The Great NHS Heist* documentaries
- Join/follow the **National Health Action Party**: www.

nhaparty.org
- Exert pressure on the **Labour Party**
- Write to your local **MP**
- If you are a doctor then be active in your **BMA** local division and the grassroots **Doctors for Progress** movement
- Get involved with the nursing **Bursary or Bust** campaign
- Consider joining the Unite/Medical Practitioners' Union (**MPU**)
- Arrange a local meeting with **38 Degrees** for concerned people in your area
- Attend local **Keep Our NHS Public** meetings: www.keepournhspublic.com
- Affiliate to the umbrella group **Health Campaigns Together**

When Aneurin Bevan was sceptically asked how long the NHS would survive, he is thought to have said, **'As long as there's folk with faith left to fight for it.'**

The biggest weapon in this fight will be you - patients and the public. Thousands of people are using GP surgeries and hospitals every day. If we can get the word out to them of what is happening, then the momentum of a national campaign to save the NHS will be unstoppable.

The historic events of recent years are testimony to what people power can achieve. When people have united in solidarity and spoken truth to power then paper tigers, whether media moguls or Middle East dictators, have often crumbled. May you live in interesting times as they say.

We started with a few questions about the NHS. I have tried to answer them. But now it's my turn. I have one question for Theresa May:

WHO GAVE YOU PERMISSION TO BREAK UP OUR NHS AND SELL IT OFF?

Afterword - How to Save the NHS in 5 Easy Steps

1. Value health and social care professionals

An incoming progressive government should reverse the new junior doctors' contract in order to show that it values their work. It should also reinstate the student nursing bursary in order to encourage nursing applications, which have dropped precipitously. Unlike most students, student nurses are working on hospital wards hence why they should be entitled to bursaries. Similarly, social care workers should have their pay and conditions drastically improved considering that they are not paid for time in between visits for example.

2. Reverse privatisation

It is paramount that privatisation is reversed by repealing the HSCA, ending private sector outsourcing and reversing the market. A publicly funded, run, owned and accountable NHS is far more cost-efficient than the current marketised system.

Fortunately, the legislation for much of this already exists - it is called the NHS Reinstatement Bill. The Conservatives have no intention of touching these proposals with a barge pole despite promises that the NHS is safe in their hands. Jeremy Corbyn and John McDonnell are two of its earliest signatories. It has cross-party support from Labour, SNP and Green MPs. However, vigilance will be necessary to ensure that this legislation is not watered down by vested interests.

The HSCA must be repealed in its entirety and not just the Section 75 competition regulations as some seem to be indicating. Labour shadow health secretary Jonathan Ashworth is inconsistent, speaking of ending privatisation and repealing the HSCA yet, in the same speech to Unison in 2017, also stating that he will retain its integral structures - CCGs - as well as outsourcing. This approach is sickeningly familiar from the Clintonite and Blairite playbook of triangulation; signalling to the left whilst moving to the right in order to reassure vested interests. It is therefore imperative that the Parliamentary Labour Party aligns with the leadership in the fight to restore a public NHS.

3. Abolish PFI

Scandalous PFI debts are saddling hospitals. As you will recall, the original capital cost of over 100 PFI hospitals is around £11.5 billion. The repayments could cost up to £80 billion. This differential of tens of billions will be siphoned off to banks, financial companies, construction and facilities management firms instead of being spent on patient care. To add insult to injury, PFI profits often end up offshore in order to enable tax avoidance.

The recent demise of construction giant Carillion has been followed by the collapse of Capita's market value: both firms having built huge empires by providing outsourced services to public authorities. These initial tremors might be the canary in the coal mine. Profit warnings have been issued for other government contractors, such as Interserve.

Haringey Council's public-private partnership with construction and property giant Lendlease appeared on the brink of collapse after Labour's National Executive Committee intervened. Similar schemes across London and the country have been plagued with controversy. Jeremy Corbyn hailed the potential halt of the Lendlease scheme as a victory for municipal socialism over what are often deemed to be unaccountable corporate interests.

One of the wider issues - a recurrent theme since the aftermath of the 2007-8 crash and consequent litany of financial sector scandals - has been the clean bill of health given by auditors. Big four accountancy firms, such as KPMG and PwC, were present at the inception of PFI. And it now looks like they might be brought in to administer the last rites. Inevitably, this raises pressing questions as to what kind of resolution entangled vested interests might propose.

So what can be done about PFI? It is often said that Scotland has turned its back on PFI. In reality, Scotland has adopted an alternative model of public-private partnership through Scottish Futures Trust. The difference is that this is not off the government's books in the same way that PFI is. As a result, Scotland's budget deficits breached EU limits - a reminder that the Maastricht Treaty paved the way for PFI by setting limits on public spending within a monetarist framework.

PFIs are complex, financial instruments and the answer needs to be carefully thought out. PFI companies are already arming themselves for the prospect of a Corbyn government as has been recently reported. John Laing Infrastructure Fund updated shareholders that it would expect 86 per cent of the value of its PFI contracts to be compensated in the event that they were taken back into public ownership. This figure may certainly prove to be questionable.

Furthermore, the catch-all of commercial confidentiality has erected a firewall. Professor Allyson Pollock has stated that contracts have to be made transparent in order to be scrutinised. Ultimately, though, the fiat of government legislation is sufficient to overhaul PFI. A spokesperson for The People versus Barts Health PFI campaign group informs me that nationalisation of the Special Purpose Vehicle (SPV) would be necessary, or perhaps even outright termination of the contracts.

Shadow chancellor John McDonnell has adopted the most progressive solution - nationalisation of the SPV. Simply centralising the debt might still mean taxpayers forking out billions as profits for PFI consortia, whilst buy-outs would be an expensive commercial solution. Labour MP Stella Creasy's suggestion of a windfall tax on PFI companies is a Blairite solution to a Blairite problem; ensuring the status quo remains intact.

PFI goes right to the heart of neoliberal orthodoxy. It means that we need to reverse financialisation. Public services, housing, education, health and social care must be restored as social goods not as financial instruments for investors. We also need to move beyond the concept of austerity and the neoliberal doctrine that public spending must be curtailed. Massive public investment is clearly needed as an alternative to the disastrous legacy of PFI. Quantitative easing was used to bail-out the big banks in the aftermath of the financial crisis. So why not have People's Quantitative Easing, dreamt up by economist Richard Murphy and previously endorsed by McDonnell, to build homes, create climate jobs and invest in public services?

We need to examine ideas, such as Modern Monetary Theory. Labour's 2017 manifesto was fully costed and operated within the present framework of balancing the books. The national conversation cannot be changed overnight. However, it would be a fatal error if a Corbyn government attempted to implement a progressive agenda operating within this fiscal envelope. It is essential to understand that sovereign governments with a currency-issuing monopoly can spend sufficiently to meet the productive capacity of the economy.

4. Ensure proper funding

Approximately £40 billion in efficiency savings combined with freezing the budget means that the NHS is undergoing the biggest funding squeeze since its inception. Unsurprisingly, it is hitting the buffers.

In other words, this is a manufactured crisis due to deliberate policies. NHS spending remains significantly less than France, Germany or Holland; less than the EU average and well below the US. By increasing spending, we would only be matching other advanced economies.

Funding is a fundamental issue but only once privatisation has been halted. Otherwise the budget is merely a funding stream diverted as profits for private companies masquerading under the NHS logo. Virgin has won almost £2 billion worth of NHS contracts since 2010. In fact, it won £1 billion of contracts in 2016 alone.

May recently announced an extra £20 billion NHS funding package by the year 2023 as a birthday present. The announcement was timed to coincide with the health service celebrating 70 years. However, it is worth paying attention to the small print in order to interrogate this birthday bonanza. The extra £20 billion set for five years' time would still fall short of the 4% historical average increase in funding per annum. The funding package also comes with strings attached to a US style model of accountable/integrated healthcare with the danger of carving up health and social care multi-billion 10-15 year contracts for private healthcare and insurance companies. Beware of Greeks bearing gifts especially when that present is a Trojan horse for privatisation.

It is important to highlight that the NHS debate has been largely contained to the issue of funding with little discussion of the juggernaut of privatisation. Liberal voices presenting themselves as defenders of the NHS - ranging from media outlets to MPs - refuse to talk about privatisation afraid of taking on the power of multinational corporations and financial capital. This is certainly convenient for the government to say the least.

The removal of the market from the NHS would solve many of its problems and release tens of billions of pounds. The introduction of market forces and private companies into healthcare is proven to escalate costs and fragment services both here and across the world. The internal market accounts for between £4.5-£10 billion of the annual budget. The extensive market accounts for billions more.

The pernicious myth that the NHS is unaffordable and unsustainable must be busted. This is merely the language of corporate lobbyists and is a fairy-tale of PR and spin. The NHS unaffordability narrative was largely created by the privatisation lobby and their media cheerleaders. In reality, public healthcare systems are the most cost-effective.

5. Legislate against corporate capture

The unrelenting focus on former health secretary Jeremy Hunt was a convenient distraction. Jeremy Hunt became a lightning rod for the medical profession's dissatisfaction and the wider public's disgruntlement with an NHS pushed to breaking point. Personnel change cannot halt the juggernaut of privatisation. His new replacement Matt Hancock is likely to be no better. Hancock has already waded into controversy over £32,000 in donations from Neil Record – the current chairman of right-wing think-tank the Institute of Economic Affairs (IEA) appointed in 2015 after seven years on its board.

The IEA describes itself as the original free market think-tank. It was instrumental in the emergence of neoliberalism – the free market orthodoxy entailing deregulation, financialisation, privatisation and shrinking the public sector. Its head of health and welfare Kristian Niemietz is in favour of NHS privatisation and its replacement with an insurance system. Kate Andrews from the IEA recorded a video (to coincide with the NHS birthday) for BBC Newsnight arguing for the overhaul of the NHS.

Hancock voted in favour of the Lansley Health and Social Care Act 2012. He also voted in favour of removing limits on how much foundation trust hospitals could earn through private patient income. According to *The Times*, the world famous Royal Marsden NHS foundation trust is now making 45% of its income from private patients and other non-NHS sources.

Privatisation is driven by the political, corporate and financial elite. A huge apparatus of private healthcare and insurance corporations, management consultancies, accountancy firms and big banks all stand to benefit. As a result, big banks – caught red-handed in one nefarious scandal after another – have financed (and in some cases effectively own) NHS hospitals. They are profiting from over £300 billion of PFI debt for the entire UK. Big three management consultancies help write health policy. Big four accountancy firms are paid millions to restructure NHS services through a massive programme of cuts and closures.

The creation of chains of super hospitals and networks of GP surgeries paves the way for potential private equity and hedge fund takeovers. Economies of scale are certainly more enticing and lucrative for corporate takeovers and private investors. One look at social care in which chains of nursing and residential homes are owned by private equity and hedge funds resulting in wealth extraction from captive public services is a chilling forecast of the direction of travel for the NHS.

Don't be fooled, the replacement of Jeremy Hunt with Matt Hancock merely represents a changing of the guard.

The first thing necessary is to define what a twenty-first century truly public NHS would look like. Renationalisation is not sufficient even if the original model of doctors and matrons on hospital boards was markedly preferable to the market model. The NHS should not simply be run either by the state or the market. It should be run by healthcare professionals, patients and communities whilst being taxpayer funded. A truly public NHS would also encompass democratic policy and decision-making. More stringent legislation is required to deal with lobbying, donations, the revolving door, regulatory capture and other strategies of corporate capture.

However, a Corbyn government could be contained by corporate and financial interests. It would be in danger of suffering the same ignominious fate as Greece's Syriza, which was crushed by global capital. Burgeoning local campaigns, mobilising in response to cuts and closures, will need to be joined up into a mass movement. Mass movements change history when broad-based bottom up coalitions combine with enlightened, progressive top-down leadership.

It is up to each and every one of us to save our NHS.

Reading List

Books

NHS SOS - Jacky Davis and Raymond Tallis (eds.), Oneworld, 2013

The Plot Against the NHS - Colin Leys and Stewart Player, The Merlin Press, 2011

The End of the NHS - Allyson Pollock, Verso, 2018

Papers

Opening the oyster: the 2010-11 NHS reforms in England - RCP Clinical Medicine 2012 Vol 12, No2:128-32 Lucy Reynolds & Martin McKee

Health and Social Care Bill 2011: a legal basis for charging and providing fewer health services to people in England - BMJ 17/3/12 Allyson Pollock, David Price, Peter Roderick

References

Introduction

1   Preface, *The Plot Against the NHS* by Colin Leys and Stewart Player. The Merlin Press - 2011.

2   'The Ultimate Indignity of the A&E Closures', *Daily Mail* 23/11/13.

3   Ken Clarke quote from *Never Again? The Story of the Health and Social Care Act* by Nicholas Timmins.

Chapter 1

1   Karen Bloor et al., 'NHS Management and Administration Staffing and Expenditure in a National and International Context', March 2005 as referenced in Health Committee Fourth report on Commissioning 18/3/10.

2   'The billions of wasted NHS cash no-one wants to mention' - Caroline Molloy, OpenDemocracy 10/10/14.

Chapter 2

1   *The Plot against the NHS*, Chapter 1 on Tim Evans and the concordat.

2   *The Plot Against the NHS*, Chapter 1 on ISTCs.

3   BMA pamphlet 'Look After Our NHS' - February 2010 - original source Department of Health & Parliament Health Select Committee 2007-8.

4   'NHS privatisation keeps on failing patients', *The Guardian* 15/8/14.

5   'PFI contracts: the full list', *Guardian* datablog (Source HM Treasury) 5/7/12.

6   'Must we sack teachers to pay for £320 plug sockets', *Daily Telegraph* 25/1/11.

7   'Private Finance Initiative: hospitals will bring taxpayers 60 years of pain', *Daily Telegraph* 24/1/11.

8   'Financial crunch tips NHS towards £1bn deficit', *The Guardian* 16/9/14.

9   Health & Social Care Information Centre for numbers and salaries.

10 BMA: 'How much does it cost to train a doctor in the United Kingdom?' and 'The cost of surgical training' by the Association of Surgeons in Training & Royal College of Surgeons in England.

11 Papworth Hospital NHS Trust Website.

12 'NHS: what we give and what we get', *BBC News* 11/4/06.

13 'Must we sack teachers to pay for £320 plug sockets', *Daily Telegraph* 25/1/11.

14 'PFI contracts: the full list', *Guardian* datablog (Source HM Treasury) 5/7/12.

15 Barts Health interest rates taken from Sir Richard Sykes, chairman of Imperial College NHS Trust as quoted in 'Charing Cross Sell-Off vital to avoid disastrous PFI deal' by Ross Lydall 26/9/14.

16 'Private Finance Initiative: hospitals will bring taxpayers 60 years of pain', *Daily Telegraph* 24/1/11.

17 Innisfree website.

18 'How PFI is crippling the NHS', *The Guardian* 29/6/12.

19 'PFI schemes will cost every household nearly £400 next year', *Telegraph* 28/4/11.

20 New Economics Foundation Mythbusters, 'The private sector is more efficient than the public sector' April 2013.

21 Report: 'New PFI initiative will saddle NHS trusts with worse debts than before', *The Independent* 26/11/14.

Chapter 3

1   See *The Plot Against the NHS* for more on GP contracts, outsourcing of OOH care, APMS contracts, integrated care and foundation trusts.

2   'Serco investigated over claims of "unsafe" out of hours GP

service', *The Guardian* 25/5/12.

3   'Services provider established by outsourcing giant Serco overcharged NHS by millions', *The Independent* 27/8/14.

4   'Former Harmoni clinician warns of "dangerous" pressure on appointments', *The Guardian* 18/12/12.

5   See *The Plot Against the NHS*, Chapter 3 for more on OOH outsourcing.

6   'The NHS is on the brink: can it survive till May 2015?', *The Guardian* 9/5/14.

7   'Do we have too many hospitals?', *BMJ* 13/2/14 2014;348:g1374 John Appleby.

8   See *The Plot Against the NHS*, Chapter 2 on payment by results.

9   'The billions of wasted NHS cash no-one wants to mention', Caroline Molloy, OpenDemocracy 10/10/14.

10 'Planning for closure: the role of special administrators in reducing NHS hospital services in England' - *BMJ* 2013;347:f7322 13/12/13.

11 'Serco: the company that is running Britain', *The Guardian* 29/7/13.

12 'Lockheed and the Future of Warfare', *New York Times* 28/11/04.

13 See *The Plot Against the NHS* on UnitedHealth & Netcare.

14 Fortune website.

15 'UnitedHealth Sues Insurance Commissioner', *USA Today* 11/7/14.

16 'Calls for greater disclosure on NHS chiefs' meetings with private US health insurer', *The Guardian* 30/8/14.

17 'The firm that hijacked the NHS', *Mail on Sunday* 12/2/12.

Chapter 4

1   'Andrew Lansley takes post advising drugs firm involved in dispute with NHS', *The Guardian* 16/11/15.

2   'The privatising cabal at the heart of our NHS' - Tamasin

Cave, OpenDemocracy, 31/3/15.

3   Hansard, Health Care Providers debate, 10/11/03 vol 413 cc133-4W.

4   'NHS boss Stevens and the TTIP "trade" lobbyists who threaten our NHS', OpenDemocracy 23/10/14.

5   'Medtronic, UnitedHealth Group want to export US health care', *Star Tribune* 26/9/11.

6   'Simon Stevens' switch to NHS is "like Arsenal signing Mesut Ozil", *The Guardian* 25/10/13.

7   'Is Simon Stevens really the right person to run the NHS?', *The Independent* 24/10/13.

8   'Simon Stevens: NHS will be "unaffordable" without radical reforms', *The Independent* 10/3/15.

9   'Spending breakdown reveals how NHS England cash flowed to private firms', *The Guardian* 27/11/14.

10 'Behind closed doors: how much power does McKinsey wield' - *BMJ* 2008; 337:a2673 12/5/12.

11 'Health trusts spend £300m on private consultants', *The Guardian* 20/8/10.

12 'NHS spending on management consultants doubles under the Coalition', *Daily Telegraph* 9/12/14.

13 'Accenture escapes £1bn penalty for NHS walk-out', *The Register* 29/9/06, originally published on Kablenet.

14 Nick Seddon material from 'This can't go on' by Andrew Robertson of Social Investigations for OpenDemocracy 13/5/13.

15 'Selling-Off NHS for profit', *Daily Mirror* 17/11/14 and 'NHS Privatisation: Compilation of financial & vested interests', Social Investigations Blog 18/2/12.

16 'Companies with links to Tories "have won £1.5bn worth of NHS contracts"', *The Guardian* 3/10/14.

Chapter 5

1   Department of Health factsheets 'Overview of the Health &

Social Care Act' 30/4/12.

2 'Can we afford the NHS in future?' *BMJ* 2011;343:d4321 12/7/11 John Appleby.

3 'Why the health service needs surgery by Andrew Lansley', *Telegraph* 1/6/11.

4 'Financial crisis is inevitable in the NHS', *BMJ News* 10/5/14.

5 'Rises in healthcare spending: where will it end?' *BMJ* 2012;345:e7127 1/11/12 John Appleby.

6 'Why the US healthcare system is failing, and what might rescue it' - *BMJ* 2012;344:e3052 9/5/12.

7 'The NHS belongs to the people: a call to action', NHS England 11/7/13.

8 'New Tory-appointed NHS boss admits: "I don't use the NHS"', *Daily Mirror* 30/10/11.

9 'A Guide to the Reforms', Keep Our NHS Public.

10 'DH to hand over billions of pounds underspend to Treasury', *Pulse Magazine* 21/8/13.

11 'A Decade of Austerity?', Nuffield Trust 3/12/12.

12 'A productivity challenge too far?' - *BMJ* 2012;344:e2416 19/6/12 John Appleby.

13 'NHS finances: the tanker en route for the iceberg' - *BMJ* Editorials 10/5/14.

14 See *The Plot Against the NHS*.

15 'NHS is the world's best healthcare system', *The Guardian* 17/6/14.

16 2011 Commonwealth Fund report and 'Mirror, Mirror on the Wall, 2014 Update: How the US Health Care System Compares Internationally'.

17 'Coalition health bill will undermine NHS, says OECD thinktank', *The Guardian* 23/11/11.

18 'London NHS hospital trust Barts Health losing £2m a week', *The Guardian* 17/7/13.

19 'Mass closure of NHS walk-in centres is fuelling winter crisis', claim campaigners. *The Guardian* 7/1/18.

20 'Why A&E departments are fighting for their life', *The Guardian* 14/1/14.

21 'NHS trusts are enmeshed in private provision - as buyers and suppliers', *The Guardian* 18/12/12.

22 'Hospitals under pressure as "bedblocking" hits record levels', *The Guardian* 28/11/14.

23 'NHS care at home for elderly and disabled quietly slashed by a third', *Daily Telegraph* 14/1/14.

24 A Guide to the Reforms, Keep Our NHS Public.

25 'Does poor health justify NHS reform?' - *BMJ* 2011;342:d566 28/1/11 John Appleby.

26 'Better data means better care in the NHS', *The Guardian* 2/12/12.

27 'British Social Attitudes Survey - how what we think and who thinks it has changed', *The Guardian* 17/9/12.

28 'Britons are more proud of their history, NHS and army than the Royal Family', Ipsos Mori 21/3/12.

29 'Coalition health bill will undermine NHS, says OECD thinktank', *The Guardian* 23/11/11.

Chapter 6

1 'David Cameron is accused of a "sham listening exercise" on NHS reform after links to lobbyist are revealed', *The Guardian* 25/11/12.

2 *Never Again: The Story of the Health & Social Care Act*, Nicholas Timmins.

3 'Equity and Excellence: Liberating the NHS', White Paper - 12/7/10.

4 'It is the only change management system you can actually see from space - it is that large', Sir David Nicholson, former NHS chief executive.

5 'David Cameron is accused of a "sham listening exercise" on NHS reform after links to lobbyist are revealed', *The Guardian* 25/11/12.

6   'This can't go on', Andrew Robertson of Social Investigations for OpenDemocracy 13/5/13.

7   'The day they signed the death warrant for the NHS', *Daily Telegraph* 25/7/11.

8   'It's already happened', James Meek, London Review of Books 22/9/11.

9   'Cameron: The First Cut', Anthony Seldon, Institute for Public Policy Research 30/9/14.

10   'It's already happened', James Meek, London Review of Books 22/9/11.

11   'Opportunities Post Global Healthcare reforms', Apax Partners October 2010.

12   *Never Again: The Story of the Health & Social Care Act*, Nicholas Timmins.

13   'What we know so far…the Health & Social Care Act 2012 at a glance' - BMA April 2012.

14   'Health and Social Care Bill 2011: a legal basis for charging and providing fewer health services to people in England' *BMJ* 2012;344:e1729, Allyson Pollock, David Price and Peter Roderick 8/3/12.

15   Monitor board from www.gov.uk website.

16   'Key Tory MPs backed call to dismantle NHS', *The Observer* 16/8/09.

17   'You must stop A&E cuts: Powerful lobby of 140 top doctors sign damning letter to PM', *Daily Mail* 7/10/12.

18   'NHS being "atomised" by expansion of private sector's role, say doctors', *The Guardian* 6/1/13.

19   'Bain Capital buys majority stake in Plasma Resources UK', *The Guardian* 18/7/13.

20   '"Arms race" over £5bn in NHS work', *Financial Times* 29/7/13 and '£5.8bn of NHS work being advertised to private sector', *Financial Times* 29/7/14.

21   'Private firms on course to net £9bn of NHS contracts', *The Guardian* 18/7/14.

22   'Rise in bailouts as more hospitals overspend on budgets',
     The Guardian 22/7/14.
23   'NHS privatisation fears deepen over £1bn deal', *The
     Guardian* 26/7/13.
24   'NHS cancer care could switch to private contracts in £700m
     plans', *The Guardian* 2/7/14.
25   Keep Our NHS Public Parliamentary Briefing 21/2/13.
26   'The NHS at 65: chaos, queues and mounting costs', *The
     Guardian* 5/7/13.
27   'A healthy market? Lack of transparency raises doubts about
     NHS commissioning' - *BMJ* 2013;347:f7115 4/12/13.
28   'The billions of wasted NHS cash no-one wants to mention',
     Caroline Molloy, OpenDemocracy 10/10/14.
29   'The NHS at 65: chaos, queues and mounting costs', *The
     Guardian* 5/7/13.
30   'NHS spent £1.8m on abandoned George Eliot competition',
     Health Service Journal 7/10/14.
31   'The billions of wasted NHS cash no-one wants to mention',
     Caroline Molloy, OpenDemocracy 10/10/14.
32   'More than a third of GPs on commissioning groups have
     conflicts of interest' - *BMJ* 14/3/13 2013;346:f1569.
33   'NHS approaches equity groups for services takeover',
     Financial Times 3/11/13.
34   'International arms firm Lockheed Martin in the frame for
     £1bn NHS contract', *The Independent* 19/11/14.
35   'Calls for greater disclosure on NHS chiefs' meetings with
     private US health insurer', *The Guardian* 30/8/14.
36   '16 thoughts on "American corporate foxes to ransack NHS
     henhouse in £3-5 bn privatisation"', Upper Calder Valley
     Plain Speaker blog, 15/11/15.
37   'Private Sector consortium wins commissioning support
     services contract' - *Health Investor UK*, 8/12/15.
38   'Private patient income soars at NHS trusts', *The Guardian*
     19/8/14.

39 'NHS trusts chasing private patients at expense of waiting lists, warns Labour', *The Observer* 16/11/14.

40 'World's largest private healthcare company HCA plans expansion into NHS', *The Independent* 14/6/13.

Chapter 7

1 'Margaret Thatcher's role in plan to dismantle welfare state revealed', *The Guardian* 28/12/12.

2 Ridley Report (Final Report of the Nationalised industries Policy Group), p15, 30/6/77.

3 'Opening the Oyster: the 2010-11 NHS reforms in England' - RCP Clinical Medicine 2012 Vol 12, No2:128-32 Lucy Reynolds & Martin McKee.

4 'Britain's biggest enterprise', Oliver Letwin and John Redwood for the Centre for Policy Studies 1988.

5 'Letwin: "NHS will not exist under Tories"', *The Independent* 6/6/04.

6 'The Health of Nations', Madsen Pirie for the Adam Smith Institute 1988.

7 *Never Again: The Story of the Health & Social Care Act*, Nicholas Timmins.

8 'NHS reforms our worst mistake, Tories admit', *The Times* 13/10/14.

9 'The truth about Sustainability and Transformation Plans', Stewart Player, 25/5/17.

Chapter 8

1 'Wards in a fifth of NHS hospitals face the axe', *Daily Telegraph* 5/10/12.

2 'District nurse numbers under pressure', BBC News, 20/11/17.

3 'NHS trusts are enmeshed in private provision - as buyers and suppliers', *The Guardian* 18/12/12.

4 'Integration? The opposite is true in Jeremy Hunt's NHS',

The Guardian 11/10/12.

5   'GPs put the squeeze on access to hospital care' - *BMJ* 10/7/2013 2013;347:f4432.

6   'Devon - the canary in the NHS coalmine?', OpenDemocracy 4/12/14.

7   '£207m debt at PFI-saddled hospital trust "should be written off"', *Daily Telegraph* 29/10/12.

8   'Private Finance Initiative: hospitals will bring taxpayers 60 years of pain', *Telegraph* 24/1/11.

9   'Lewisham Hospital: Appeal Court overrules Jeremy Hunt', *BBC News* 29/10/13.

10 'Planning for closure: the role of special administrators in reducing NHS hospital services in England' - *BMJ* 13/12/132013;347:f7322 Allyson Pollock, David Price et al.

11 'PFI hospital crisis: 20 more NHS trusts "at risk"', *Daily Telegraph* 26/6/12.

12 'Shaping a Healthier Future Pre-consultation Business Case', Appendix C, p.15.

13 'NHAP condemns massive cuts in West London Hospitals', National Health Action Party statement 21/2/13.

14 'Royal baby NHS trust to slash NHS beds and boost private income', *Evening Standard* 12/8/14.

15 'Health boss pulls out of £120,000 taxpayer-funded "study tour"', *Evening Standard* 28/11/14.

16 'The list of 66 A&E and maternity units being hit by cuts', *Daily Telegraph* 26/10/14.

17 'Lewisham is just the start of hospital protests to come', *The Guardian* 25/1/13.

18 'NHS strike: Staff begin biggest strike in 30 years over 1% pay row', *The Independent* 13/10/14.

19 'Hospitals and fire services to be run "outside the public sector"', *Daily Telegraph* 14/12/14.

20 'Mutual ownership: privatisation under a different name?' *BMJ* 21/8/14 2014;349:g5150 by Martin McKee.

Chapter 9

1   'Junior doctors are victims of an NHS that's broken beyond repair', *Daily Telegraph* 4/11/15.

2   'Strike won't cure sick NHS', *The Sunday Times* 8/11/15.

3   'Increased mortality associated with weekend hospital admission: a case for expanded seven day services?' Freemantle, N et al. *BMJ* 5/9/15.

4   'Secret documents reveal official concerns over "seven-day NHS" plans', *The Guardian* 22/8/16.

5   'Five go to war with the government', *The Independent* 8/9/16.

6   'Labouring under the delusion of secrecy - the clandestine McDonnell policy review', Health Policy Insight Editorial, 28/6/16.

7   'Labour health advisers angered by John McDonnell's parallel group', *The Guardian* 30/6/16.

8   'Why I had to leave Corbyn's dysfunctional shadow cabinet by Heidi Alexander', *The Guardian* 19/8/16.

9   'Revealed: Ed Miliband's Pfizer insider in the shadow Cabinet', *Daily Telegraph* 10/5/14.

10   'Owen Smith backed big pharma over use of cheaper drugs by NHS in 2010', *The Guardian* 20/7/16.

11   'Owen Smith backed big pharma over use of cheaper drugs by NHS in 2010', *The Guardian* 20/7/16.

12   'Public supportive of moves to increase choice but government must do more to make it a reality' - King's Fund Press Release 31/10/05.

13   'Owen Smith on the Iraq war, working as a lobbyist and the role of the private sector in the NHS', Wales Online 10/5/06.

14   Select Committee on the Long-term Sustainability of the NHS, Corrected oral evidence: 12/7/16.

15   'Only a Royal Commission will get us talking sensibly about the NHS', *Daily Telegraph* 16/12/15.

Chapter 10

1 '"Accountable Care" - the American import that's the last thing England's NHS needs', Stewart Player, OpenDemocracy 1/3/16.

2 '"Accountable Care" - the American import that's the last thing England's NHS needs', Stewart Player, OpenDemocracy 1/3/16.

3 'Accountable care models contract: proposed changes to regulations', Department of Health, 11/9/17.

4 'Outsourcing firm and US healthcare insurer team up to run STP', *BMA News* 24/8/17.

5 'One in six A&E departments at risk of closure or downgrade', *The Guardian* 6/2/17.

6 'Spring NHS crisis even worse than winter, "Black Thursday" data shows', *Daily Telegraph* 12/5/16.

7 'What caused the spike in mortality in England and Wales in January 2015?' Lucinda Hiam, Danny Dorling, Dominic Harrison, Martin McKee. *Journal of the Royal Society of Medicine*. Volume: 110 issue: 4, page(s): 131-137 1/4/17.

8 'Rise in mortality in England and Wales in first seven weeks of 2018', Hiam, L. & Dorling, D. *BMJ* 14/3/18.

9 Watkins J, Wulaningsih W, Da Zhou C, et al 'Effects of health and social care spending constraints on mortality in England: a time trend analysis', *BMJ Open*, Volume 7 Issue 11, 2017.

10 '600 GP practices could close by 2020, warns RCGP', *PharmaTimes* 20/9/16.

11 'Mass closure of NHS walk-in centres is fuelling winter crisis, claim campaigners'. *The Guardian* 7/1/18.

12 'NHS plan for 7,500 GP practices to become 1,500 "superhubs" revealed', *Daily Telegraph* 16/3/17.

13 '"Accountable Care" - the American import that's the last thing England's NHS needs'. Stewart Player, OpenDemocracy, 1/3/16.

14 'Fears of "two-tier NHS" as GPs allow fee-paying patients to jump the queue', *The Guardian* 8/2/17.

15 'Royal Free breached UK data law in 1.6m patient deal with Google's DeepMind', *The Guardian* 3/7/17.

16 'Hospital records of all NHS patients sold to insurers', *Daily Telegraph* 23/2/14.

17 'Surge in privatisation threatening free NHS treatment, unions say', *The Guardian* 8/2/16.

18 'Tory plans for NHS privatisation released during parliamentary recess', Alex Scott-Samuel, *BMJ* 5/8/16.

19 'Guy's Hospital opens £160 million cancer centre', *Evening Standard* 26/9/16.

20 'The Game Changer: US Health Group Eyes Up NHS contracts', *The Independent* 9/2/15.

21 'US firms look to capitalise as NHS becomes increasingly privatised', *The Guardian* 8/2/16.

22 'The Americanisation of the NHS, happening right here, right now', Public Matters blog 30/8/17.

23 'Patients with long term conditions can hold own budgets from 2015', *BMJ News* 19/7/14.

24 'More hospitals could be privately operated in NHS shakeup, says review', *The Guardian* 5/12/14.

25 'Revealed: All new GP contracts will be thrown open to private providers', *Pulse Magazine* 18/8/14.

26 'The real force behind the NHS Act - the EU/US trade agreement', Linda Kaucher, OpenDemocracy 19/2/13.

27 'This transatlantic trade deal is a full-frontal assault on democracy', George Monbiot, *The Guardian* 4/11/13.

28 'Trade secrets: will an EU-US treaty enable US big business to gain a foothold?' - *BMJ* 5/6/13 2013;346:f3574.

29 'The NHS will fail us so long as we look on it as a market', *The Guardian* 8/8/13.

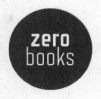

CULTURE, SOCIETY & POLITICS

Contemporary culture has eliminated the concept and public
figure of the intellectual. A cretinous anti-intellectualism
presides, cheer-led by hacks in the pay of multinational
corporations who reassure their bored readers that there is no
need to rouse themselves from their stupor. Zer0 Books knows
that another kind of discourse – intellectual without being
academic, popular without being populist – is not only possible:
it is already flourishing. Zer0 is convinced that in the unthinking,
blandly consensual culture in which we live, critical and engaged
theoretical reflection is more important than ever before.
If you have enjoyed this book, why not tell other readers by
posting a review on your preferred book site.

Recent bestsellers from Zero Books are:

In the Dust of This Planet
Horror of Philosophy vol. 1
Eugene Thacker
In the first of a series of three books on the Horror of Philosophy,
In the Dust of This Planet offers the genre of horror as a way of
thinking about the unthinkable.
Paperback: 978-1-84694-676-9 ebook: 978-1-78099-010-1

Capitalist Realism
Is there no alternative?
Mark Fisher
An analysis of the ways in which capitalism has presented itself
as the only realistic political-economic system.
Paperback: 978-1-84694-317-1 ebook: 978-1-78099-734-6

Rebel Rebel
Chris O'Leary
David Bowie: every single song. Everything you want to know,
everything you didn't know.
Paperback: 978-1-78099-244-0 ebook: 978-1-78099-713-1

Cartographies of the Absolute
Alberto Toscano, Jeff Kinkle
An aesthetics of the economy for the twenty-first century.
Paperback: 978-1-78099-275-4 ebook: 978-1-78279-973-3

Malign Velocities
Accelerationism and Capitalism
Benjamin Noys
Long listed for the Bread and Roses Prize 2015, *Malign Velocities* argues against the need for speed, tracking acceleration as the symptom of the ongoing crises of capitalism.
Paperback: 978-1-78279-300-7 ebook: 978-1-78279-299-4

Meat Market
Female Flesh under Capitalism
Laurie Penny
A feminist dissection of women's bodies as the fleshy fulcrum of capitalist cannibalism, whereby women are both consumers and consumed.
Paperback: 978-1-84694-521-2 ebook: 978-1-84694-782-7

Poor but Sexy
Culture Clashes in Europe East and West
Agata Pyzik
How the East stayed East and the West stayed West.
Paperback: 978-1-78099-394-2 ebook: 978-1-78099-395-9

Romeo and Juliet in Palestine
Teaching Under Occupation
Tom Sperlinger
Life in the West Bank, the nature of pedagogy and the role of a university under occupation.
Paperback: 978-1-78279-637-4 ebook: 978-1-78279-636-7

Sweetening the Pill
or How We Got Hooked on Hormonal Birth Control
Holly Grigg-Spall
Has contraception liberated or oppressed women? *Sweetening the Pill* breaks the silence on the dark side of hormonal contraception.
Paperback: 978-1-78099-607-3 ebook: 978-1-78099-608-0

Why Are We The Good Guys?
Reclaiming your Mind from the Delusions of Propaganda
David Cromwell
A provocative challenge to the standard ideology that Western power is a benevolent force in the world.
Paperback: 978-1-78099-365-2 ebook: 978-1-78099-366-9

Readers of ebooks can buy or view any of these bestsellers by clicking on the live link in the title. Most titles are published in paperback and as an ebook. Paperbacks are available in traditional bookshops. Both print and ebook formats are available online.

Find more titles and sign up to our readers' newsletter at http://www.johnhuntpublishing.com/culture-and-politics

Follow us on Facebook
at https://www.facebook.com/ZeroBooks

and Twitter at https://twitter.com/Zer0Books